Regional Anaesthesia in Children

Regional Anaesthesia in Children

Claude Saint-Maurice

M.D., Professor
Dept of Anaesthesia
Hopital Saint Vincent de Paul
Paris, France

Ottheinz Schulte Steinberg

M.D.D.A. (McGill)
Former Chief of Dept. of Anaesthesia.
Kreiskrankenhaus Starnberg, Academic Teaching
Hospital of the Ludwig-Maximilians-
University Munich, Germany

Edward N. Armitage

M.B., B.S., F.F.A.R.C.S.
Language coordinator
Consultant Anaesthetist
Royal Alexandra Hospital for Sick Children,
Brighton, England

Lennart Håkansson

Coordinator

Poul Buckhöj

Medical artist

Foreword by

Philip R. Bromage

M.B.B.S., F.F.A.R.C.S., F.R.C.P.(C)

APPLETON & LANGE/MEDIGLOBE
Norwalk, Connecticut/San Mateo, California/Fribourg, Switzerland

3

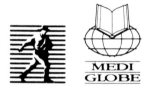

Library of Congress Cataloging-in-
Publication Data

Regional anaesthesia in children / [edited by]
Claude Saint-Maurice, Ottheinz Schultz
Steinberg, Edward N. Armitage; Lennart
Håkansson, coordinator; Poul Buckhöj, medical
artist; foreword by Philip R. Bromage.
    p.   cm.
  ISBN 0–8385–8304–0
  1. Conduction anesthesia in children.
I. Saint-Maurice, Claude.   II. Steinberg,
Ottheinz Schultz.   III. Armitage, Edward N.
[DNLM: 1. Anesthesia, Conduction--in infancy
& childhood.   WO 300 R3352]
RD84.R418   1990
617.9'64--dc20
DNLM/DLC
for Library of Congress   90–229
                                       CIP

Printed by
KIN KEONG PRINTING CO PTE
LTD SINGAPORE

4

Foreword

Since the introduction of curare in the 1940's, it has not been easy for anesthetists to convince themselves and their surgical colleagues that regional anesthesia still has value when muscle relaxants have made general anesthesia so simple, reliable and relatively trouble-free.

However, with the passage of time and the persistence of a few enthusiasts, enough evidence has accumulated to vindicate regional anesthesia in two important areas. First, superb and prolonged pain relief; and second, the ability of skillfully applied deafferentation to preserve and even restore function once the reflex inhibitory effects of pain are overcome. Most of this work has been done in adults, and the specialty has been slow to apply the benefits of regional anesthesia to children, where the margin for error is less, and where the effects are more difficult to measure in little patients too young to comprehend what is happening. But the qualitative results are very persuasive. The doubter has only to spend a day in a pediatric recovery ward of orthopedic patients under regional anesthesia to be convinced by the aura of gentle alertness and calm, in contrast to the dramatic difference from a ward full of children returning to a world of pain and distress after conventional general anesthesia. Moreover, freedom from the need for postoperative ventilatory support is a major advantage, especially in premature infants with immature lungs and central control systems.

It is a great honor to be asked to write a foreword to this volume. After more than twenty years of innovative clinical investigation with epidural analgesia in children Professeur Saint-Maurice and Dr. Schulte-Steinberg have assembled a team of European collaborators to present a wide spectrum of pediatric regional anesthesia in practical handbook form. Much of this material is of value to the occasional pediatric anesthetist. However, the authors' have dealt very fairly with the difficulties and potential dangers of major spinal blockade, such as thoracic epidural blockade, in young children. With increasing regionalization of pediatric surgical services, it is likely that the more demanding techniques will become increasingly confined to pediatric units specializing in the types of major surgery where these complicated block find their most appropriate application.

The authors pragmatic approach to pediatric regional anesthesia will ensure a warm welcome for their practical handbook among the anesthetic profession with primary interests in the operating room or in acute pain management during the perioperative period.

Philip R. Bromage

M.B.B.S., F.F.A.R.C.S., F.R.C.P.(C)

Contributors

T.C.Kester. Brown
Royal Children´s Hospital
Flemmington Road - Parkville
MELBOURNE VICTORIA
Australia

Paolo Busoni
Ospedale Pediatrico
A. Meyer
Via Luca Giordano 13
FIRENZE
Italy

Marie Madeleine Delleur
Hospital Saint Vincent De Paul
Department of Anaesthesia and Intensive Care
74 Avenue Denfert Rochereau
75014 PARIS
France

Anne Marie Dubousset
Hopital Bicetre
Departement d´ anesthesiologie
78 Rue Du General Leclerc
94270 Le KREMLIN-BICETRE Cedex
France

Catherine Esteve
Department of Anaesthesia and Intensive Care
Hospital Saint Vincent De Paul
74 Avenue Denfert Rochereau
75014 PARIS
France

Elisabeth Giaufre
Hopital Saint Joseph
Chirurgie pediatrique
26 Boulevard de Louvain
F-13008 MARSEILLE
France

Jean-Luc Hody
Clinique Sainte Anne
14 Place de la Vaillance
B-1070 ANDERLECHT
Belgium

Jean Xavier Mazoit
Hopital Bicetre
Departement d´ anesthesiologie
78 Rue Du General Leclerc
94270 Le KREMLIN-BICETRE Cedex
France

Michel Meignier
Hotel Dieu
Unit of Pediatric Anaesthesia
F-44035 NANTES Cedex 01
France

Isabelle Murat
Hospital Saint Vincent De Paul
Department of Anaesthesia and Intensive Care
74 Avenue Denfert Rochereau
75014 PARIS
France

Claude Saint-Maurice
Department of Anaesthesia and Intensive Care
Hospital Saint Vincent De Paul
74 Avenue Denfert Rochereau
75014 PARIS
France

Ottheinz Schulte Steinberg
Dietrichweide 7
D-8130 STARNBERG 2
Germany

Contents

I. Basic principles

II. Techniques

III. Pain management

IV. Uncommon diseases and special problems

Index

I. Basic principles

General principles and benefits

Ottheinz Schulte Steinberg

Regional blocks in children are valuable techniques both for use in the awake child and for supplementing general anaesthesia. However, certain safeguards have to be observed.

1. The anaesthetist must already have acquired experience and dexterity with regional anaesthesia in adults before he employs the techniques in children. It is very important that he has developed a feeling for the needle as it traverses different tissues, such as ligaments and aponeuroses, and meets obstacles such as cartilage and bone. The sensation transmitted to the hands as the loss of resistance sign is elicited must be familiar. This is particularly important because the size of the spaces being located can be very small in young children and fascial layers are thinner and more difficult to recognise. Skill and experience are therefore prerequisites, but it is still advisable to start with the simple blocks when first applying regional anaesthesia to children.

2. There are important anatomical differences between the small child and the adult, and the anaesthetist must be aware of these if he is to avoid complications.

3. The dosage of a local anaesthetic drug obviously varies with the weight of the child and the site of application of the drug, but other factors have also to be taken into account. For example, age influences the absorption and plasma concentrations of local anaesthetics. Tracheal administration in children below the age of 3 years tends to result in higher plasma concentrations than in older children and adults, even when equal doses are given on a weight-for-weight basis. Also, protein binding of local anaesthetics in children and enzyme activity affecting their degradation are different from adults (1,2). On the other hand, when diazepam or a general anaesthetic are given separately or together, the threshold for convulsions is increased considerably.

..In summary, great care must be taken when the total dose of local anaesthetic is being calculated. The calculation must include the topical dose as well as the dose given for the block. Fortunately, satisfactory blocks can be obtained with comparatively low concentrations of drug in small children, so if a large volume is required for a successful block, this does not necessarily mean that a large mass of drug has to be given.

4. Consideration has to be given to individual drug profiles so that the choice of agent is appropriate to the operation and to the age and mental development of the child. A long-acting agent such as bupivacaine is suitable for a long operation or one which causes considerable pain in the immediate postoperative period. Short-acting agents are appropriate for short procedures which do not cause much postoperative pain. High concentrations of local anaesthetic drugs which produce motor block are unsuitable if the primary object of the block is to produce analgesia, and a drug such as etidocaine which produces a powerful motor block even in low concentration should be avoided altogether. Young children may become quite upset and restless if they cannot move their legs due to a caudal induced with a high concentration of drug. With lower concentrations, satisfactory analgesia can be obtained, yet motor power to the lower limbs remains unaffected. Paraesthesiae do still occur, but they seem to be better tolerated and are only admitted by the child on direct questioning (3). If motor block is specifically required for a particular operation, it can be produced by the addition of adrenaline to the local anaesthetic drug, by using a higher concentration of drug or by using etidocaine.

5. Skin infection in the area of needle and catheter insertion is an absolute contraindication to regional anaesthesia.

6. In recent years there has been an increasing appreciation of the value of catheters in regional anaesthesia. Whereas their use was almost entirely limited to epidural and caudal blocks,

they have now been found suitable for peripheral blocks such as the axillary and intercostal. Not only does a catheter enable the analgesia to be prolonged, but it allows the local anaesthetic to be deposited in a localised area which may not be readily accessible to the needle. An indwelling catheter is, in effect, a foreign body and there is the possibility that it may become infected unless it is inserted under aseptic conditions. There should therefore be distinct indications for its use.

7. Coagulation disorders preclude all central blocks unless they can be corrected beforehand. This is particularly important when a block is being considered for a premature baby. Central blocks are contra-indicated in patients who are receiving chemotherapeutic agents for the treatment of malignancies. Such agents lead to vascular fragility and this may predispose to bleeding when a needle or catheter is introduced into the epidural or subarachnoid space.

8. Before performing a block, the anaesthetist must have a clear strategy concerning the technique, the equipment, the drugs and the dosage. He must also make sure that his assistant is well versed in the procedure and is capable of administering the general anaesthetic while the block is being performed. Good organisation prior to the procedure helps to avoid delays, emergencies and excitement.

9. Close monitoring with regional anaesthesia is just as important as with general anaesthesia since the clinical condition can change very rapidly, particularly in the premature and the newborn, regardless of the type of anaesthetic given.

Monitoring should always start with clinical observation of the patient. The colour of the skin can give valuable information about the state of oxygenation, peripheral perfusion and circulating blood volume, and it may enable hypoxia and hypovolaemia to be detected. A precordial or oesophageal stethoscope is a simple and reliable device for monitoring cardiac rate and rhythm throughout the anaesthetic and particularly during the injection of the local anaesthetic and the onset of the block. It also monitors respiration. Since increases in cardiac rate and respiration are the usual responses to surgical stimulus, the stethoscope can provide the anaesthetist with a good indication of the extent and adequacy of the block. A blood pressure cuff of appropriate size is mandatory. The acoustic pulse monitor or the rate monitor of the electrocardiograph (ECG) can be used to pass cardiovascular information to the rest of the team. The ECG also enables the anaesthetist to recognise at once any arrhythmias and changes in rate. This is of particular importance at the time of injection of the test dose. Local anaesthetic agents containing adrenaline are often used as test doses because, if a needle or catheter has accidentally been placed intravascularly, changes in rate or rhythm will be seen within a minute of the injection. This is a better indication of the position of the catheter than an aspiration test, which is not infrequently negative even when the catheter lies in a vein.

The small child loses heat under general anaesthesia and, since central blocks cause vasodilatation, they tend to increase this heat loss. Oesophageal or rectal temperature probes are therefore required to monitor body core temperature. The need for other, more sophisticated monitoring is dictated by the type of surgery to be performed and by the condition of the child. The reader is referred to the standard paediatric textbooks.

10. It is sometimes claimed that the addition of a regional block to a general anaesthetic submits the child to the risks of two techniques instead of one. There is no reason why this should be so. Indeed, it is probably more accurate to claim that the combination of regional and general anaesthesia conveys the benefits of both techniques to the child. The over-riding considerations are the safety of the child, the reduction of the stress of surgery and the prevention of postoperative pain. The advantages of regional anaesthesia in attaining these objectives are listed below.

Benefits

1. Analgesia provided by the regional block reduces the amount of general anaesthesia required and thus allows it to be maintained at lighter levels . This has several consequences. First, the lactic acidosis which results from a general anaesthetic, especially halothane, is reduced (4), as is the incidence of postoperative vomiting. The latter is further reduced by the fact that little or no opioids are required for analgesia in the postoperative period. Second, the child

wakes soon after the end of surgery so the potentially hazardous recovery period is shortened. Third, intake of oral fluids can begin earlier, and stand a better chance of being retained, so that the detrimental metabolic effects of anaesthesia and surgery are minimised.

2. Undesirable autonomic reflexes, causing laryngospasm and cardiac arrhythmias, are common during stimulating surgery of the perineum and foreskin, and deep general anaesthesia is required to obtund them. Regional block eliminates these reflexes and allows lighter levels of general anaesthesia to be used.

3. Muscle relaxation can be obtained if a suitable local anaesthetic is used in an appropriate concentration. Etidocaine and the higher concentrations of bupivacaine provide profound relaxation. Thus, non-depolarising muscle relaxants become unnecessary and there is then no need for the use of reversal drugs or for post-operative ventilation which is sometimes required when respiratory insufficiency follows the administration of a muscle relaxant. This is an important factor in the premature and newborn baby in whom the neuromuscular junction is immature.

4. Immobilisation of a limb after delicate surgery is simplified if the child is pain-free and if there is some residual motor block. A certain amount of oedema inevitably follows surgical trauma, but it tends to be less if a regional block has been used. This is probably because venous drainage to the area is improved.

5. In adults, modification of the stress response, more rapid recovery and a shorter stay in hospital have been observed following regional block. Similar findings have now been reported in children (5,6,7,8).

6. In cases with a family history of malignant hyperpyrexia a regional block may be the technique of choice. Both ester- and amide-linked local anaesthetic agents appear to be safe in this condition (9).

7. Hypotension and urinary retention are rarely observed after regional block in children. In the presence of a central block, renal perfusion is assumed to be dependent on peripheral blood pressure, so children with renal disease are good candidates for such a block.

8. Intra- and post-operative bleeding is reduced under neural blockade (8).

9. Incarcerated hernias can often be reduced with ease under caudal block. This obviates the need for immediate surgery with its inherent danger of aspiration from a full stomach, and enables the operation to take place under optimal conditions.

10. Premature and formerly premature babies suffer from bronchopulmonary dysplasia long after they have recovered from the respiratory distress syndrome. They tolerate anaesthesia badly and have a high incidence of respiratory complications, notably apnoeic attacks, in the postoperative period. When such babies require abdominal surgery (for example, for herniorrhaphy), a central block such as a spinal has the advantage that perfect analgesia and relaxation can be obtained without recourse to general anaesthesia or interference with the respiratory tract, and the incidence of respiratory complications is reduced (10). The same may be true for caudal anaesthesia (11).

11. Open anaesthetic systems with relatively high gas flows are commonly used for administering general anaesthesia to children. These systems are wasteful and cause pollution since the scavenging of exhaled gases is difficult. A regional block, used in conjunction with general anaesthesia, reduces this problem, and when used as the sole anaesthetic technique, it eliminates it entirely.

References

1. Brown TCK and Fisk GC (1979) Anaesthesia for Children.Blackwell Scientific Publications, Oxford, London, Edinburgh, Melbourne,
2. Eyres RE, Kidd J, Oppenheim R and Brown TCK (1978) Anaes Intens Care 6:243
3. Armitage EN (1985) Regional anaesthesia in paediatrics, Clinics in Anaesthesiology 3:560
4. Reinauer H und Hollmann S (1966) Der Einfluß der Narkoseart auf den Gehalt an Adeninnukleotiden, Lactat und Pyruvat in Herz, Leber und Milz der Ratte. Anaesthesist 15:327
5. Giaufre E, Morisson-Lacombe G and Rousset-Rouviere B (1983) L'anesthesie caudale en chirurgie pediatrique. Chir Pediatr 24:165

6. Giaufre E, Conte-Devolx B, Morisson-Lacombe G, Boudouresque F, Grino M, Rousset-Rouviere B, Guilleame V and Oliver C (1985) Anesthesie peridurale par voie caudale chez l'enfant, Etude des variations endocriniennes. La Presse Medicale 14:201

7. Murat I, Wacker J, Esteve C, Nahoul K, Saint-Maurice C (1988) The efect of continuous epidural anaesthesia on plasma cortisol levels in children. Can Anaesth J 35:20

8. Tozbikian H (1988) Continous thoracic Epidural Blockade for Rectus Thoracoplasty in Children. Regional Anesthesia 13:25

9. Boninsegni R, Salerno R, Giannotti P, Andreuccetti T, Busoni P, Santoro S, Forti G (1983) Effects of surgery and epidural or general anaesthesia on testosterone, 17-hydroxyprogesterone and cortisol plasma levels in prepubertal boys. J Steroid Biochem 19:1783

10. Harnik EV, Hoy GR, Potolicchio S, Stewart DR and Siegelman RE (1986) Spinal anesthesia in premature infants recovering from respiratory distress syndrome. Anesthesiology 64:95

11. Spear RM Deshpande JK ,and Maxwell LG (1988) Caudal Anesthesia in the Awake High Risk Infant. Regional Anesthesia 13:24

History

Ottheinz Schulte Steinberg

Spinal Anaesthesia

Although we tend to think of paediatric regional anaesthesia as being a relatively modern development, it does in fact date from the earliest pioneering days. Bier (1), in his original paper on spinal anaesthesia published in 1899, described the effects in an 11 year old boy! In 1900, Bainbridge (2) followed with a similar report on 5 children under the age of 8 years, and by 1901, further reports had appeared on children between the ages of three months and six years (3). The technique remained popular, particularly in Canada, throughout the 1930s and 1940s. Junkin (4) in 1933 and Robson (5) in 1936 had reported on spinal anaesthesia for thoracic surgery in children, and Koster (6) in 1928 had even recommended it for surgery of the head and neck. The place of spinal anaesthesia was sufficiently established for Leigh and Belton (7) to be able to include it in their book "Paediatric Anesthesia" in 1948, and Lemmon and Hager (8) in 1944 were the first to use continuous spinal anaesthesia in a series of 33 children.

However, the 1950s saw improvements in general anaesthesia, with the development of better equipment and new drugs, particularly the muscle relaxants. As a result, spinal anaesthesia for children lost its popularity. Nevertheless, areas remain in which general anaesthesia is not entirely satisfactory. New ideas about operative stress and the metabolic changes which occur during and after surgery are now better appreciated, and the ever-present possibility that a child will need postoperative ventilation after receiving muscle relaxants is well recognised. These and other factors have rekindled interest in regional anaesthesia, and although the simplicity of the caudal block and the introduction of the epidural have challenged the popularity of the spinal in paediatric practice, papers on the subject do still sporadically appear.

Epidural Anaesthesia

Epidural anaesthesia in children was first described by Sievers (9) in 1936 and the idea was revived in 1951 by Schneider (10) who reported over 6.500 children, 25% of whom were babies, operated on under lumbar epidural block. Both these workers used the technique for urological procedures. Ruston (11,12,13) introduced continuous lumbar anaesthesia in 1959. His papers show that he used epidural block in infants and children for more than 12 years during which time he published 170 cases. He found that sick children requiring surgery for acute conditions such as intussusception did well, but he also used continuous epidural block for extensive abdominal procedures lasting up to 6 hours and he lists hemihepatectomy, repair of omphalocoele, Hirschsprung's disease and removal of pelvic tumour among his cases. Prior to the block and during surgery, all these patients were intubated and received light general anaesthesia with nitrous oxide, oxygen and halothane 0.25%. Intermittent, small doses of succinylcholine were given "to paralyse the diaphragm during its repair or to relax spasm caused by accidental movement of the child's head, which caused it to buck on the tube." From his comments, it is quite obvious that he used a modern technique combining regional and general anaesthesia. Despite this, Ruston remained a lone prophet. His methods were not generally accepted and were sometimes actually condemned.

In 1971, Isakob and colleagues (14) published a report of thoracic epidural block in children for postoperative analgesia. They inserted an epidural catheter between T3 and T7 at the end of thoracic operations and maintained the analgesia for two to three days.

The safety of spinal and epidural anaesthesia is borne out by a report by Zeng Gang from China, on 10.000 cases in small children without a single neurological or infectious complication. There were less than 10 total spinals (15).

Caudal anaesthesia

The caudal approach to the epidural space was described in children by Campbell (16) in 1933. Further reports appeared by Spiegel (17) in 1962 and by Fortuna (18) in 1967, followed by many others in more recent years. In 1984, Schulte-Steinberg and Busoni (19) showed that caudal catheters could be advanced to lumbar and even thoracic levels in young infants and small children.

Other regional techniques

Brachial plexus block in children was described by Farr (20) in 1920, but it was 28 years before the paper by De Pablo and colleagues appeared, in which they reported 3.000 cases (21). Accardo and Adriani (22) described the axillary approach in children in 1949, and Winnie (23) the interscalene technique in 1970.

Although the nerve stimulator had been described by Perthes as long ago as 1912, it was Aizenberg (24) who opened the door for the wider application of peripheral nerve blocks under sedation or general anaesthesia by demonstrating its value in the very young patient.

Intravenous regional anaesthesia has not been widely adopted in children, but in 1971, Carrell and Eyring (25) reported its use for the treatment of fractures. The youngest child in the series was 3 years.

Summary

In adults, regional anaesthesia has undergone an impressive renaissance based on the availability of safe, long-acting local anaesthetic agents and better understanding, and management, of the cardiovascular changes which occur during a block. The re- introduction of the nerve stimulator has cleared the way for the safe performance of peripheral blocks in young patients under general anaesthesia. These developments have been accompanied by the realisation that general anaesthesia and regional block can be advantageously combined. This is of particular benefit in paediatric practice because the block can be performed under ideal conditions and, since only very light levels of general anaesthesia are subsequently needed, postoperative recovery is rapid as well as painless. This is important because current opinion favours the performance of minor paediatric surgery on an outpatient basis whenever possible (3).

References

1. Bier A (1899) Versuche über die Cocainisierung des Rückenmarks Dtsch Ztschr f Chir 51:361
2. Bainbridge WB (1900) Analgesia in children by spinal injection with a report of a new method of sterilization of injection fluid. Medical Record 58:937
3. Armitage EN (1985) Regional anaesthesia in paediatrics. Clinics in anaesthesiology 3:535

4. Junkin CI (1933) Spinal anesthesia in children. Canad Med Assoc J 28:51

5. Robson CH (1936) Anesthesia in Children. Am J Surg 34:468

6. Koster H (1928) Spinal anesthesia in head and neck surgery. Am J Surg 5:571

7. Leigh MD and Belton MK (1948) Pediatric anesthesia, New York. The Macmillan Co 121

8. Lemmon WT and Hager Jr HG (1944) Continuous spinal anesthesia: Observations on 2000 cases. Ann Surg 120:129

9. Sievers R (1936) Peridurale Anaesthesie zur Cystoskopie beim Kind Arch Klin Chir 185:359

10. Schneider, Leipzig Kinderklinik (1951) Peridural Anaesthesie im Kindesalter. Z Urol Chir 76:704

11. Ruston FG (1954) Epidural anaesthesia in infants and children. Can Anaesth Soc J 1:37

12. Ruston FG (1957) Epidural anaesthesia in pediatric surgery. Anesth Analg 36:76

13. Ruston FG (1964) Epidural anaesthesia in paediatric surgery: Present Status at the Hamilton General Hospital. Can Anaes Soc J 11:12

14. Isakob YF, Geraskin BI and Koshevnikov VA (1971) Long term peridural anesthesia after operations on the organs of the chest in children. Grudnaja Chirurija 13:104

15. Zhen-Gang Zhan (1986) Poster: Spinal, epidural and supportive basal anaesthesia in their use at Beijing Children's Hospital. First European Congress of Paediatric Anaesthesia, Rotterdam, Aug 27-30th. Book of Abstracts 132

16. Campbell MF (1933) Caudal anesthesia in children. J Urol 30:245

17. Spiegel P (1962) Caudal anesthesia in pediatric surgery: A preliminary report. Anesth Analg 41:218

18. Fortuna A (1967) Caudal analgesia: A simple and safe technique in paediatric surgery. Br J Anaesth 39:165

19. Schulte Steinberg O and Busoni P to be published

20. Farr RE (1920) Local anesthesia in infancy and childhood. Arch Pediatr 37:381

21. De Pablo JS and Diez-Mallo J (1948) Experiences with 3000 cases of brachial plexus blocks: Its dangers: Report of a fatal case. Ann Surg 128:956

22. Accardo NJ and Adriani J (1949) Brachial plexus block: A simplified technique using the axillary route. South Med J 42:920

23. Winnie AP (1970) Interscalene brachial plexus block. Anesth Analg 49:455

24. Aizenberg VL (1972) The technique of regional anesthesia of the extremities in combination with nitrous oxide general anesthesia in children. Vestn Khir 108:88

25. Carrell ED and Eyring EJ (1971) Intravenous regional anesthesia for childhood fractures. J Trauma 11:30

Anatomy

Paolo Busoni

General considerations

The following discussion is limited to the peculiarities of the anatomy of children, to the differences between children and adults, and to the ways in which these differences affect the use of regional anaesthesia in children. For full details and information, the reader is referred to standard anatomical textbooks.

The changes of form which take place during human growth are well-defined. The cephalad end of an embryo differentiates first and grows more rapidly in utero than the caudad end. This is known as the antero-posterior gradient. Thus, a newborn child has a relatively large head attached to a medium-sized body with diminutive legs and feet. As growth proceeds, this gradient is reversed and although the head continues to grow, it does so slower than the rest of the body so that, relatively, its size decreases (3)(Fig. 1). When the anaesthetist performs central blocks in children, from the newborn to the adolescent, he has to pay close attention to these changes in body size.

The depth of important structures varies according to the age and size of the patient. Ligaments and fascia are thinner in children and easier to penetrate, but they are more difficult to identify unless short-bevelled, or comparatively large, needles are used. In small children, the nerves are thinner and myelination is incomplete. These factors mean that diffusion and penetration of local anaesthetic can occur easily, and satisfactory blocks can be achieved with lower concentrations of drug than would be required in adults.

Fig. 1. Changes in body proportion from birth to adulthood.

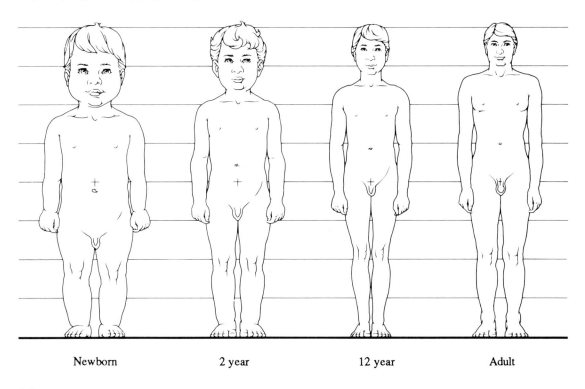

Newborn   2 year   12 year   Adult

However, the same factors result in slower rates of nerve conduction, and this must be borne in mind when the effectiveness of a block is being assessed (2). For example, grimacing or crying as a response to a stimulus may take up to 5 seconds to appear. A similar immaturity of the autonomic nervous system has been found and it may explain why hypotension is rarely seen in children even after extensive central blocks.

Age, weight and length (height) can be used for calculation of the dose required to anaesthetize one spinal segment. Schulte Steinberg has shown that all these parameters correlate well with dosage and spread.

In calculating the dosage required in thoracic epidurals, the author has used his experience obtained with continuous caudal anaesthesia (p. 88) in which age was found to be the most accurate predictor. However, weight is the most practical for purposes of calculation.

Anatomy of the spine

Knowledge of the development of the spinal cord and spine is necessary for our understanding of the anatomical features in the child.

The foetal cord initially occupies the entire length of the spinal canal, but after the fourth month of intrauterine life, it no longer extends into the lower part of the canal (Fig. 2). This is due to the fact that the spinal column begins to grow in length more rapidly than the cord itself (3,4).

Ossification centres

Three primary ossification centres appear in the cartilaginous vertebrae at about the tenth foetal week. They consist of a single osseous nucleus in the body, two nuclei in the arch and one in each pedicle. The fusion of the ossification centre in the body with the centre in the arch takes place between the third and sixth years. The two bony centres in the arch fuse posteriorly, and complete the bony neural arch during the first two postnatal years.

Secondary ossification centres begin to appear in the annular cartilages shortly before puberty in females, and somewhat later in males. The secondary vertebral ossification centres (superior articular processes, transverse processes, spinous processes and inferior articular processes) appear at approximately 16 years and fuse with their

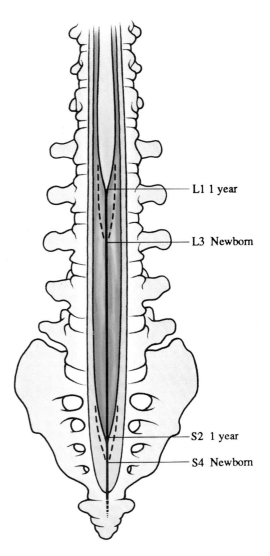

Fig. 2. The central nervous system, comparison of a child 4 months of age and adult

respective processes at about 25 years (5).

In the sacrum, ossification of the central part of the bodies of the first three vertebrae commences at about the eighth or ninth week of foetal life, and between the sixth and eighth months ossification of the laminae and lateral masses takes place. The bodies of the sacral vertebrae are separated from each other by intervertebral discs during early life. By the eighteenth year the two

17

lowermost segments become joined together by ossification extending through the disc, and the whole process of fusion spreads upwards to the other segments. Ligamenta flava connect the upper and lower borders of the sacral vertebrae in early life; ossification takes place later between the 15th and 25th years. Complete fusion of the bone occurs between the 25th and 30th years. Therefore a needle can be inserted through the sacral interspaces toward the epidural space using the same technique as in the lumbar region. Thus a sacral intervertebral epidural block can be performed (21). The time at which the arch becomes completed by the fusion of the laminae with each other and with the body in front varies in different segments, but it does not start before the second year of life (5, 6). The spinal column in the newborn, in infants and even in children is to a large extent cartilaginous. Fusion of the laminae to each other and to the vertebral body forms the neural arch. This is completed later in the post-natal period. Thus, there is the possibility that, if needles are improperly inserted during the course of epidural and sacral blocks, they can damage these more delicate cartilaginous structures. At birth, the vertebral column forms a single, long, shallow curve, concave anteriorly. As a consequence, the spinous processes are more parallel to each other, and this facilitates epidural puncture at all levels (Fig. 3).

The average length of the spine, excluding the sacrum, is 20cm at birth. During the first and second year of life, growth is rapid and the length increases to about 45cm. Thereafter, the growth rate greatly diminishes and the length at puberty is about 50cm. The final length, attained between the 22nd and 24th years, is 60-75cm.

The relative length of the cervical and lumbar portions changes significantly during growth. At birth, the cervical spine makes up one-quarter of the total length of the spinal column, the thoracic spine one-half and the lumbar spine one-quarter. The cervical spine is proportionately longer during infancy than in later life (5). The apparent shortness of the neck in infants is due to the fullness of the cervical soft tissues. In the adult the cervical spine is reduced to one-fifth or one-sixth of the total length, while the lumbar segment is increased until it comprises nearly one-third of the whole spine.

In the cervical region, osseous fusion of the posterior ends of the neural arch in the midline is usually completed between the 4th and 6th years,

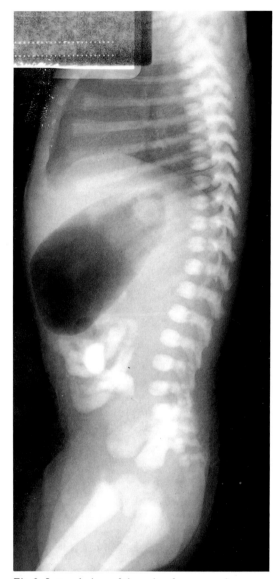

Fig.3. Lateral view of the spine from a newborn.

but it is not uncommon for the arches to remain open until later. In the Arnold-Chiari syndrome, the upper cervical canal takes the form of a funnel-shaped enlargement. The pathology consists of a herniation of the cerebellar tonsils, with swelling and posterior displacement of the medulla against the upper spinal cord.

Cervical spina bifida occulta (retardation of the closing of the neural arches of the cervical spine) is not uncommon and is often of no clinical significance (8). Errors in segmentation are not uncommonly observed in the cervical spine. Under- segmentation is more frequent than excessive segmentation. Failure of segmentation is seen in the Klippel-Feil syndrome (9) in which elevation of the scapula and webbing of the neck also frequently occur.

Cervical ribs usually cause no clinical signs, but, in a small proportion of cases, they are responsible for the so-called "cervical rib-scalene syndrome" (10). This syndrome is caused by local compression of the subclavian artery on the somatic branches of the brachial plexus and, in rare cases, on the sympathetic nerves. The arterial compression gives rise to a tingling and dull aching in the arm, and pressure on the somatic branches of the brachial plexus causes pain and paraesthesiae. If the sympathetic nerves are affected, constriction of the pupil and ptosis may result. Progressive and severe atrophy of the muscles of the hand is sometimes observed.

In the thoracolumbar region, the vertebral bodies become proportionately larger with advancing age, losing their oval shape and becoming more rectangular. In lateral radiographs, the vertebral bodies also show paired, cone-shaped, notched, shadowy defects in the middle of the anterior and posterior walls. A large sinusoidal blood space within the ossification centre is responsible for the anterior notch, while the posterior one is caused by the vertebral veins and the nutrient arteries which perforate the posterior wall of the body (11).

Pelvis

The pelvis of the foetus, infant and child is conspicuously small and funnel-shaped. During the neonatal period the vertical diameter is elongated in proportion to the lateral and sagittal diameter. At birth, the pelvic inlet tends to be more circular than in later life. The acetabular cavities are shallower and relatively larger, whereas the obturator foramina are proportionately smaller and situated close together (12).

Sacrum

This is a large triangular bone, inserted like a wedge between the two innominate bones. It makes up a large segment of the pelvic girdle during the first year, and is situated higher in relation to the ilia than in the adult (12). For this reason, the sacral hiatus in young children appears higher than expected, compared with adults (13). Once the infant assumes the erect posture, the sacrum descends between the ilia,

Fig. 4. Changes in position of iliac crest in different age groups.

Adult   ——————

Child   - - - - -

Neonate   ∙∙∙∙∙∙∙∙∙∙

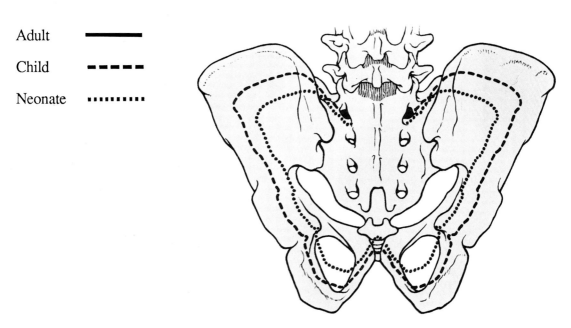

19

thus causing the promontory to become more conspicuous. Pelvic growth is rapid during the first two years, but it slows thereafter until puberty when the major sexual features appear.

Failure of segmentation between the lateral masses and transverse processes of the first sacral segment and the transverse processes of the fifth lumbar segment is responsible for the variant known as sacralisation of the fifth lumbar vertebra. In infants and children however, this condition is rarely associated with any signs or symptoms (12).

As far as surface anatomy is concerned, on average the intercristal line crosses the midline at the level of the fifth lumbar vertebra in children, and even lower, at the L5-S1 interspace, in neonates (Fig. 4.).

Spinal cord

The spinal cord gradually recedes up the spinal canal as gestation proceeds. At term, the first sacral nerve arises from the cord at the level of the first lumbar vertebra. The spinal cord itself terminates at the level of the third lumbar vertebra at term, and at the first lumbar vertebra by the end of the first year (Fig. 5).

The dural sac is extending caudad as far as the fourth sacral foramen in children, compared with the second or third in adults, and there is no cerebrospinal fluid below this level. Residual tissue from the dural sac ensheaths the filum terminale (which is thicker in the neonate than in older children) and descends to the back of the sacrum where it blends with the periosteum (14).

Fig. 5. Levels of the dural sac.
(Scientific Foundation of Paediatric. Edited by SA Davis and John Dobbing 1974, William Heineman Medical Books Ltd, London).

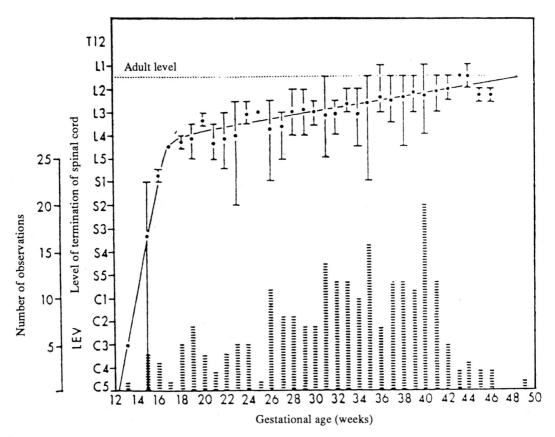

20

Cerebrospinal fluid

This fluid occupies the subarachnoid space (Fig. 6). It is formed in the choroid plexus of the lateral, third and fourth ventricles at the rate of 0.35ml.min^{-1} (500-600ml per day)(15). It circulates out of the ventricular system through the lateral fourth ventricular foramina of Luschka, and the midline fourth ventricular foramen of Magendie. 70% of the volume remains within the ventricular system. Of the remaining 30%, about 10% circulates upwards through the brainstem subarachnoid cisterns and then over the surface of the brain, and about 20% circulates downwards into the subarachnoid space of the spinal cord. Most of the fluid returns to the venous dural sinuses through the arachnoid villi which overlie the superior sagittal sinus in the midline. Infants and children who weigh less than 15kg have a relatively higher total volume of cerebrospinal fluid - 4ml.kg^{-1} compared with 2ml.kg^{-1} in adults (16).

Fig. 6.

1. *Arachnoid granulation*
2. *Dura mater (outer layer)*
3. *Dura mater (inner layer)*
4. *Subdural space*
5. *Arachnoid mater*
6. *Subarachnoid space*
7. *Superior sagittal sinus*
8. *Pia mater*
9. *Choroid plexus of 3rd ventricle*
10. *Great cerebral vein*
11. *Cisterna cerebellomedullaris*
12. *Interventricular foramen*
13. *Interpeduncular cistern*
14. *Cistern of the great cerebral vein (cisterna ambiens)*
15. *Choroid plexus of 4th ventricle*
16. *Foramen of Magendie*
17. *Superficial cerebral vein*
18. *Cerebral cortex*

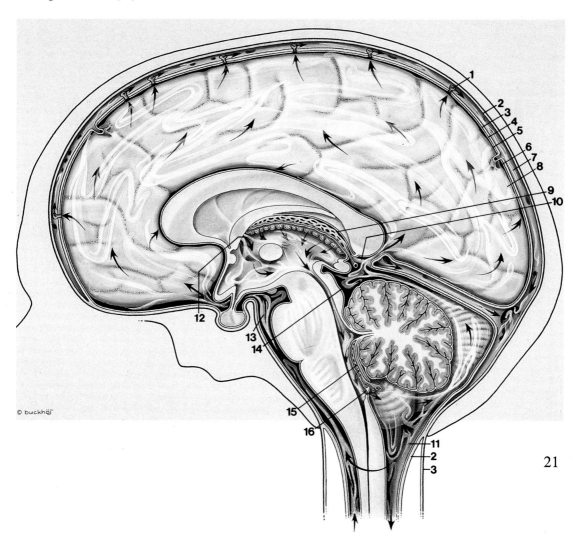

© buckhöj

21

Epidural space

This surrounds the spinal meninges and extends from the foramen magnum to the sacral hiatus. It contains nerve roots, fatty tissue, lymphatics, arteries and veins. The areolar fat is loose, with distinct spaces between the individual fat lobules, and this permits a more even distribution of injected solutions (14). The epidural space itself appears relatively large in the newborn due to the smaller amount of fatty tissue (17)(Fig. 7). Standard anatomical textbooks should be consulted for descriptions of the epidural arteries and veins. It is sufficient to observe here that, in the neonate, the anterior spinal artery is normally tortuous over the lower portion of the cord (18).

Fig. 7 Cross section of the spinal canal at the thoracic level.

1. *Posterior longitudinal ligament*
2. *Periosteum*
3. *Nerve root*
4. *Subarachnoid space*
5. *Epidural space*
6. *Pia mater*
7. *Arachnoid mater*
8. *Subdural space*
9. *Subarachnoid septum*
10. *Dura mater (inner layer)*
11. *Dura mater (outer layer)*
12. *Ligamentum flavum*
13. *Ligamentum denticulatum*
14. *Dorsal nerve root*
15. *Ventral nerve root*
16. *Dorsal root ganglion*
17. *Spinal nerve*

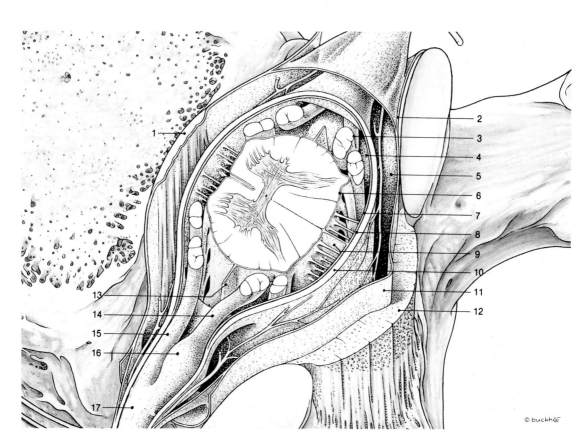

© buckhöj

The distance of the epidural space from the skin in children is of the greatest importance to the anaesthetist. It was studied at the L 3-4 level by Kosaka and colleagues (19) and at L 2-3 by Busoni (Fig. 8), and similar results were obtained in both studies. Busoni (20) found that the distance was about 10mm at birth and that it increased linearly with age according to the equation:

distance = (age in years x 2) + 10mm

so, for a three year old child, the distance of the epidural space from the skin is

(3 x 2) + 10mm = 16mm.

Application of this formula is helpful in avoiding accidental dural puncture.

Posture and movement

The spinal column, viewed from the front, can be considered as formed by two pyramids joined together at their bases, the upper one consisting of all the vertebrae from the second cervical to the fifth lumbar, and the lower one consisting of the sacrum and coccyx. Viewed from the side, the spinal column has several curves which correspond to the different regions of the column and are therefore called cervical, dorsal, lumbar and pelvic.

The cervical curve appears shortly after the head is held upright during the first year of life. The lumbar curve develops when erect posture is assumed at about the beginning of the second year and gradually becomes more prominent during the years of childhood. The cervical and pelvic curves are compensatory, or secondary, and are developed after birth in order to maintain the erect position. They are due mainly to the shape of the intervertebral discs. The dorsal and pelvic curves are the primary curves and begin to be formed in early foetal life. They are due to the shape of the vertebral bodies.

Fig. 8. Skin - epidural space distance (L2-3).

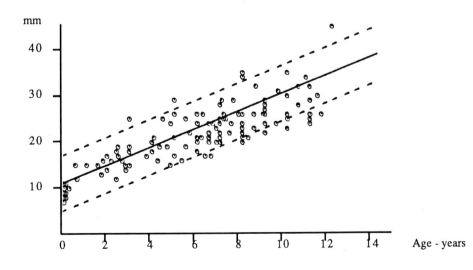

Innervation

A map of sensory dermatomes in small infants is
shown in Fig. 9.

Fig. 9. Sensory dermatomes in small infants.

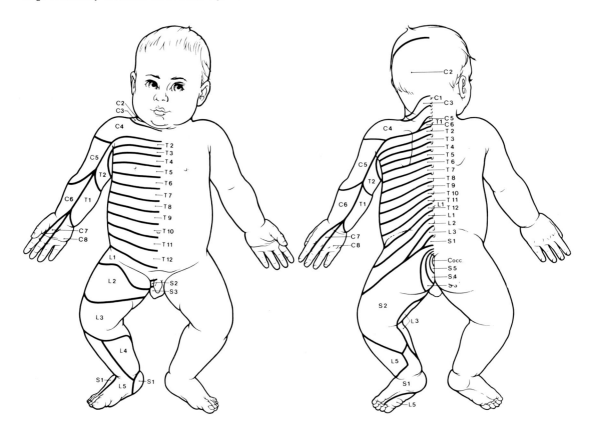

References

1. Vaughan VC (1979) Textbook of pediatrics. Edited by Nelson WE. Philadelphia-London-Toronto. Sauders pp 13-16, 26-27
2. Freeman JM (1974) Practical management of meningomyelocele. University Park Press Baltimore p 28
3. Hamilton WJ, Mossman HW (1972) Human Embryology. Cambridge. Heffer & sons
4. Gray's Anatomy (1974) Edited by Pickering Pick T. Philadelphia pp 1149-1216
5. Caffey J (1967) Pediatric X-ray diagnoses. Chicago, Year Book Medical Publishers pp 579-593, 1351-1357
6. Testut L, Latarjet A (1959) Traité d'Anatomie Humanie. Torino UTET p 85
7. Netter HF (1962) Nervous System. New York CIBA p 21-30
8. Freeman JM (1974) Practical management of meningomyelocele. Baltimore. University Park Press pp 25-29
9. Klippel M, Feil A (1912) Un cas d'absence des vertebres cervicales. Bull et Mem Soc Anat de Paris 14:185
10. Ray BS et al (1953) Cervical ribs: An analysis of findings in 57 operated cases. Buln New York Acad Med 29:60
11. Gooding CA, Neuhauser ED (1965) Growth and development of the normal vertebral body in the presence and the absence of stress. Am J Roentgenol 93:388
12. Reynolds ES (1945) The bony pelvic girdle in early infancy: A roentgenometric study. Am J Phys Anthropol 3:321
13. Mc Gown RG (1982) Caudal analgesia in children. Anaesthesia 37:806
14. Tretjakoff D (1926) Das epidurale Fettgewebe. Z Anat 79:100
15. Cutler RWP, Pae L, Galicich J et al (1968) Formation and absorption of cerebrospinal fluid in man. Brain 91:707
16. Kandt RS, Johnston M and Goldstein GW (1983) The central nervous system: Basic concept. Edited by Gregory GR New York Churchill Livingstone p 138
17. Bosenberg AT, Bland BAR, Schulte Steinberg O, Downing JW (1988). Thoracic epidural anaesthesia via the caudal route in infants and children. Anesthesiology 69:265
18. Ferguson WR (1950) Some observations on the circulation in fetal and infant spines. J Bone & Joint Surg 32-A:640
19. Kosaka Y, Sato I, Kawaguchi R (1974) Distance from skin to epidural space in children. Jpn J Anaesthesiol 23:874
20. Busoni P (1982) Lumbar extra-dural anaesthesia in newborn infants and children. ESRA meeting in Edinburgh.
21. Busoni P, Sarti A (1987) Sacral intervertebral epidural block. Anesthesiology 65:993

Physiological considerations

Elisabeth Giaufre and

Isabelle Murat

This chapter will confine itself to the ways in which central blocks and their consequences differ between children and adults. It will deal firstly with the mechanisms of action of local anaesthetics, with particular reference to epidural anaesthesia, and secondly, with the physiological consequences of central blocks.

Mechanisms of action of local anaesthetics

Action on the nerve fibre

Local anaesthetics reversibly block the initiation and propagation of the nerve action potential and thus cause both sensory and motor paralysis. Recently-introduced electrophysiological techniques have helped to elucidate this effect of local anaesthetics on the action potential (1). A transient increase in the nerve membrane's permeability to sodium is required for the initiation and

Fig. 10a. The sodium ions are in excess on the outside of the nerve membrane. Conversely, on the outside there are potasium ions in excess.

Fig 10b. During the depolarization phase. The sodium channels are open and sodium ions pass to the inside

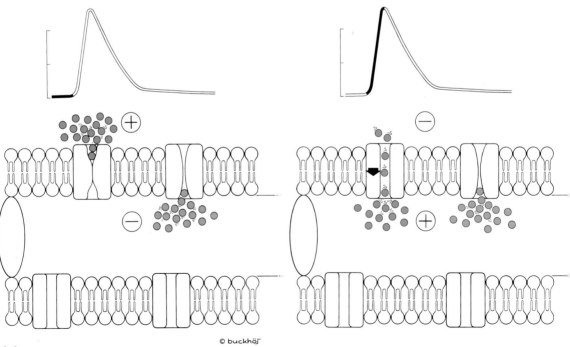

© buckhöj

conduction of an action potential and, following the studies of Hille (2), it is generally agreed that local anaesthetics reduce this permeability to sodium (Fig. 10 a-d). The unionised form of a local anaesthetic can penetrate nerve sheaths and nerve membranes, and the drug can therefore reach the sodium channels directly from the membrane or via the axoplasm. There is experimental evidence which suggests that local anaesthetics combine with a receptor in the sodium channel, and this binding prevents the passage of sodium ions through the channel. Only the ionised form of a local anaesthetic acts at the receptor. In the sodium channels themselves, there is equilibrium between the ionised and unionised forms, and this equilibrium is pH dependant (3). These aspects will be considered in more detail in the chapter on pharmacology.

Fig. 10c. During the repolarization phase. The potasium ions pass to the outside. The sodium channels are closed.

Fig. 10d. Conclusion of the action potential. The potassium and sodium ions pass back to the original position.

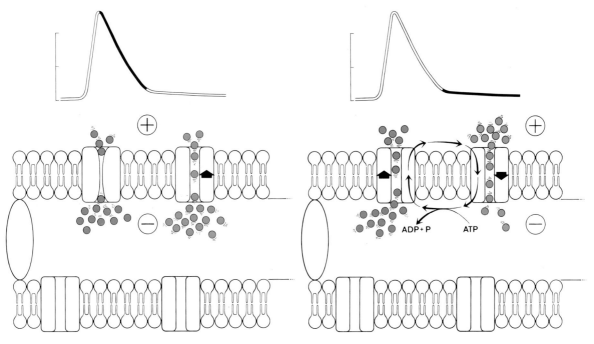

ADP + P   ATP

Differential nerve block

Ever since the work of Gasser and Erlanger in 1924 (4), it has been assumed, until recently, that conduction of impulses in small cutaneous nerve fibres is blocked earlier than in larger fibres. However, this assumption is not completely true, especially for A delta fibres (5), and it now seems that the difference between the rate at which various fibres are blocked is better explained by the distance over which the local anaesthetic has to diffuse in order to reach the fibre than by differences in the minimal concentration of drug required to block fibres of different diameters (6)(Fig. 11).

Myelinisation is incomplete at birth and continues to develop into the fourth year (7,8). The degree of myelinisation of a nerve fibre affects the rate at which it conducts an impulse. Nerve conduction velocities in the newborn are only half those of the adult due to incomplete myelinisation, but the actual conduction times for peripheral reflex arcs in the newborn are somewhat less because the conduction distances are shorter (9,10,11). The small size and in-complete myelinisation of nerve fibres in infants may account for the fact that, after epidural injection by either the caudal or the lumbar route, there is a low incidence of failed block. Patchy block also is very uncommon. Further-more, in children less than 4 years old, muscle relaxation can be obtained with low concentra-tions of local anaesthetic. 0.25% bupivacaine, for example, is sufficient to produce adequate surgical relaxation of the abdominal wall.

Fig. 11. Possible mechanism of action of epidural anaesthesia

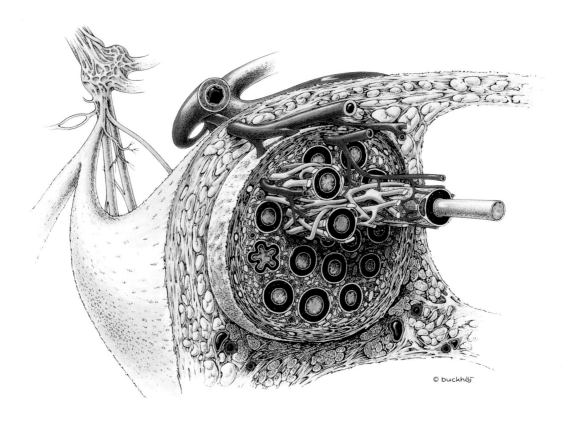

© buckhöj

Mechanism of action of epidural anaesthesia

Local anaesthetic drugs in the epidural space may act at a variety of possible sites (Fig. 12), including the spinal nerve in the paravertebral space, the dorsal root ganglion, the dorsal and ventral spinal roots and the spinal cord itself (12).

In adults, recent studies have revealed very little lateral spread when local anaesthetics are injected, indicating that the epidural space is essentially a

Fig. 12. A summary of the possible diffusion pathways of epidurally administered local anaesthetic agents to various neural structures.

1. Through dura to CSF
2. CSF to cord
3. Dural root sleeves to nerve roots and cord
4. Dural root sleeves to spinal nerve

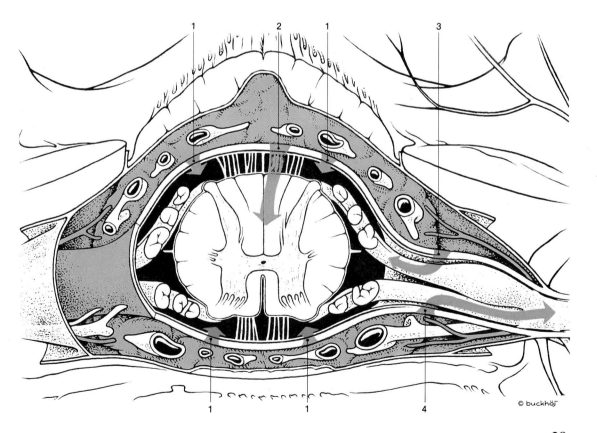

© buckhöj

closed space. Furthermore, the volume of solution injected has very little effect on its spread within the space. Ecoffey and colleagues (13) observed the effects of epidural anaesthesia in children between 3 and 36 months old. They injected 0.5% bupivacaine with adrenaline 1:200.000 in a dose of 0.75ml.kg^{-1} after a standard test dose of 0.5ml. The mean epidural spread was 12 segments (+ or - 1 segment), but the spread did not correlate with the weight of the child.

Two mechanical factors - pressure and compliance in the epidural space - may influence the outcome of an epidural block. For many years there has been lively debate about the existence and significance of the negative pressure within the epidural space (14,15).

From the anaesthetist's point of view, it is important to know that, with the exception of the caudal region, it can be identified clinically, and is more obvious in the thoracic region than the lumbar. The degree of negative pressure varies with posture and with respiration (16). However, in children, the negative epidural pressure can easily be recognised even when the child is in the supine position and receiving positive pressure ventilation.

For practical purposes, compliance is of more interest than pressure because it has a direct effect on the physical spread of injected solutions, according to the equation:

$$\text{compliance} = \frac{\text{volume of solution}}{\text{pressure of injection}}$$

In young subjects of about 20 years of age, the epidural space pressure rises sharply on injection to 8cm of water and falls rapidly, so that it is virtually back to normal after 30 seconds (17). The pattern is different in older patients. By the age of 75 years, the pressure rises on injection to 40cm of water and falls more gradually to a plateau which persists for several minutes. These differences may well be due to the fact that the nature and the extent of epidural fat varies with age. In children up to the age of 6 or 7, the epidural fat is comparatively loosely packed, whereas in the adult it is much firmer and offers greater resistance to the even spread of solutions (18).

Local anaesthetic drugs in the epidural space seem to act principally on the dorsal and ventral spinal roots (Fig. 11)

These agents can easily gain access to the roots by crossing the dura which surrounds them. As suggested above, the effect on the spinal root depends partly on the ratio of the local anaesthetic concentration to the diameter of the spinal root (19). However, the electro-physiological effect of a block (as assessed by scalp- sensory evoked potential to nerve stimulation) does not always correlate with the clinically observed extent of the analgesia (20).

Epidurally-injected local anaesthetic drugs can also enter the cerebrospinal fluid (CSF) and can then enter the spinal cord itself (Fig. 12.). However, penetration of the cord depends on the physicochemical properties of the agent. The more highly lipid soluble the drug, the greater is the penetration. Duration of action is also mainly determined by lipid solubility, though the latter has less effect on the onset of block.

In summary, the effects of local anaesthesia on a child depend to some extent on its age and state of neural development, but in general, a block is likely to extend further and be more intense than its adult equivalent. The duration of the block will depend mainly on the pharmacokinetics and pharmacodynamics of the drug, and these are considered in the chapter on pharmacology.

Pain perception

The primary aim of epidural anaesthesia is to prevent the conduction of nociceptive impulses from the surgical site to the brain, and the onset of sensory analgesia is usually the first indication of a successful block. There is very little information about the anatomical and physiological aspects of pain perception in children. Melzack and Wall (21) proposed the 'gate theory' of pain in 1965 and, more recently, Wall (22) has reappraised it. In adults, it is now conceded that pain perception is a complex process incorporating the following components:

1. The transmission of information concerning injury from the periphery to the central nervous system along peripheral nerves. The receptors at the periphery are of two types. The high threshold mechanoreceptors respond almost exclusively to intense mechanical stimulation and information from them is conducted mainly by the A

delta fibres. The polymodal receptors, as their name suggests, respond to a wide range of stimuli. Information from them is conducted by C fibres.

2. Cells in the spinal cord and 5th nerve nucleus, which are excited by injury signals. These cells are also facilitated or inhibited by input from other peripheral nerves which carry information about non-noxious events (Fig. 13).

3. Descending control systems. These modulate the excitability of cells which transmit injury signals.

Opioid receptors develop in parallel with other features of the central nervous system such as dendrites, synapses and myelinisation (23). Opioid receptors have even been found in the fetus, and their numbers increase rapidly after birth, while their affinity for opioids remains constant (24). Beta-endorphin activity in plasma from the newborn is three to four times that found in the mother or other adults (25), and beta-endorphin levels increase during the first four days of life (26). It is probable that this increased production occurs in response to changes in sensory input and to various stress stimuli resulting from the extrauterine environment. These high endorphin levels correlate with the clinical impression that neonates are relatively insensitive to pain in the first few days of life, with sensitivity increasing rapidly thereafter. It has not yet been established whether the peripheral sensory receptors are also present from birth and in sufficient numbers for adult-type pain responses to be possible, but clinical obser-vation suggests that this is a reasonable assumption.

Fig. 13. A depicts sensory afferent fibres entering the dorsal horn of the spinal column. Synaptic connections occur in the dorsal horn following which post-synaptic fibres leave the dorsal horn and travel by various pathways to the brain.

B. shows a detailed diagram of the dorsal horn with the various laminae where the numerous synaptic connections occur.

1. Dorsal column
2. Dorsal root
3. Dorsal root ganglion
4. Ventral spinothalamic fasciculi
5. Substantia gelatinosa
6. Large cutaneous fibres
7. Small cutaneous fibres
8. Visceral fibres
9. To contralateral spinothalamic tract
10. To ipsilateral spinothalamic tract

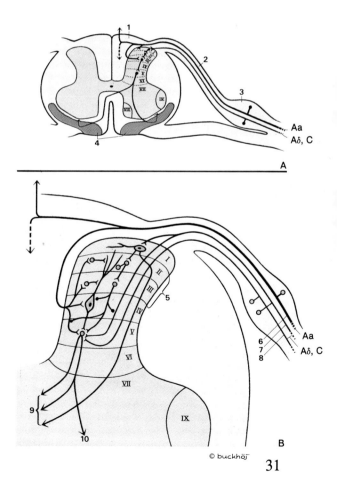

© buckhöj

31

Physiological effects of central blocks

Haemodynamic effects

These may arise from two sources. Epidural and spinal anaesthesia causes block of the lower thoracic and upper lumbar sympathetic outflow, and this results in vasodilatation of the lower limb. If the anaesthesia extends high enough, it may also cause block of the cardiac sympathetic fibres which arise from the upper four thoracic segments (Fig. 14). In adults, the main effects of a central block are a decrease in blood pressure, a decrease in cardiac output, and peripheral vasodilatation (27). These changes are related to the level of block, the amount of drug ad-ministered, the specific features of the local anaesthetic used, the addition of a vasoconstrictor to the anaesthetic solution (28), the super-imposed effect of general anaesthesia (29,30) and the age and cardiovascular status of the patient.

In children, all available studies show that epidural and spinal blocks are associated with minimal haemodynamic changes. This was first noticed, after lumbar epidural anaesthesia, by Ruston (31) in 1954, and was confirmed, after caudal anaesthesia, by Fortuna (32). More recently, Arthur (33) used thoracic epidural anaesthesia to control the systolic blood pressure after repair of coarctation of the aorta. He succeeded in preventing hypertension, but the expected decrease in blood pressure did not occur, and the patients remained very stable.

However, the haemodynamic effects of a central block do depend on the age of the child. In 1979, Dohi and colleagues (34) induced spinal anaes-thesia which produced a sensory level between T3 and T5. This caused little or no change in blood pressure or heart rate in children less than 5 years old, whereas there was a widely variable decrease in blood pressure in children older than 6 years. One of the present authors has conducted a more precise study (35)(Figs. 15 and 16) in which ASA status 1 children in three different age groups (less than 2 years, 2 to 8 years, and over 8 years) underwent epidural anaesthesia. The preinduction values of systolic blood pressure (SBP) were identical in the three groups, but as might be expected, preinduction heart rate (HR) was significantly higher in the younger children. (The decline in HR in the postnatal period seems

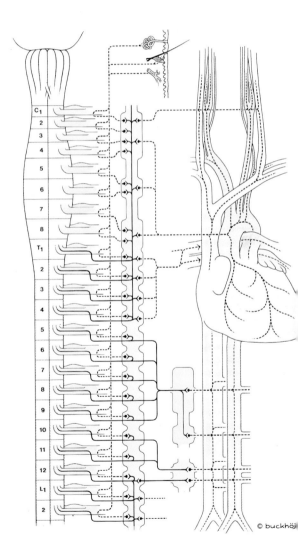

Fig. 14. Diagram showing the efferent innervation of the heart and blood vessels by the sympathetic nervous system.

to be more closely related to changes in intrinsic cardiac properties after birth than to changes in sympathetic or parasympathetic tone (36)). All the children received general anaesthesia with enflurane 1.5% and epidural block up to T6. Minimal haemodynamic changes were observed in children aged less than 2 years and in those between 2 and 8 years, whereas in children over 8 years the changes were comparable with, though less marked than, those found in adults.

It is not clear why there is a smaller decrease in blood pressure in young children. Even in young animals, after the first month of life, the neuro-hormonal control of resting blood pressure and the systemic response to autonomic agonists are identical to the adult (36,37,38). The situation may be explained by the propor-tionately smaller blood volume in the lower limbs of children, and their lower level of systemic vascular resistance

at rest (39). The practical consequence is that fluid loading and vasoactive drugs are not required prior to epidural anaesthesia in children.

Since light general anaesthesia is usually given before a regional block is performed, the combined effects of the two techniques must also be considered. Even light general anaesthesia interferes with compensatory vasoconstriction in the upper part of the body (29,30) and the halogenated agents, commonly used for main-taining general anaesthesia, exert various effects on myocardial contractility, peripheral resistance and the baroreflex response (40,41). However, low concentrations are adequate during regional anaesthesia, and most of these effects are minimal. Isoflurane seems to have less myocardial depressant action than halothane and enflurane, so it is the agent of choice when cardiovascular stability is essential (42).

Fig. 15. Change in heart rate during lumbar block I Murat et al (1987) Br J Anaesth

Fig. 16. Change in blood pressure during lumbar block. I Murat et al (1987) Br J Anaesth

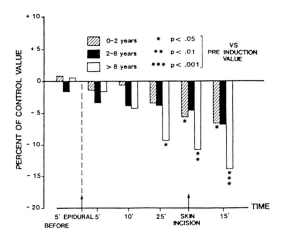

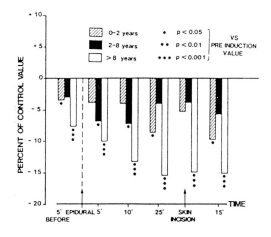

33

Effects on regional blood flow

A few studies on adult man are available with regard to regional blood flow during epidural anaesthesia (43). A 14% decrease in renal blood flow was observed in volunteers when a block to the level of T5 was produced. This occurred even though there was no significant decrease in mean blood pressure or cardiac output. On the other hand, changes in hepatic blood flow ran parallel to changes in mean arterial pressure.

The effects of epidural anaesthesia on limb blood flow have been assessed in both adults and children. In adults, a marked increase in blood flow in the lower limb is accompanied by a compensatory decrease in flow in the upper limb above the level of the block (43). In children, a pulsed Doppler technique was used to assess the relative changes in upper and lower limb blood flow following caudal anaesthesia (44). No significant change could be detected in the lower part of the body, whereas there was a significant decrease in brachial blood flow.

Effects on the respiratory system

The effect on the respiratory system of a single epidural injection of local anaesthetic depends not only on the segmental height of the block, but also on the density of block and whether motor fibres are affected as well as sympathetic and somatic ones (45,46). Apnoea is not usually a complication of a high epidural block per se, but is most often due either to an epidural dose delivered intrathecally through an accidental, unrecognised, dural puncture, or to hypoxia resulting from hypotension.

General anaesthesia with spontaneous ventilation decreases pulmonary efficiency by increasing the dead space. Intermittent positive pressure (IPPV) does not have this disadvantage. A feature of high epidural block is that reflex afferent respiratory input is reduced and the threshold of excitability rises. The consequence is that IPPV can be easily instituted without the need for supplemental drugs.

The effects of halogenated agents on the respiratory system must also be considered. Halothane anaesthesia causes an increase in respiratory frequency, a decrease in tidal volume and a decrease in ventilatory response to carbon dioxide. However, if the inspired halothane concentration remains below 1%, the changes in alveolar ventilation are minimal (47). Hatch and colleagues (48) compared a group of healthy children receiving only halothane anaesthesia with another group receiving halothane and caudal anaesthesia. Both groups were breathing spontaneously and had lower abdominal surgery. These workers concluded that caudal block and halothane anaesthesia results in more efficient ventilation during surgery by reducing the respiratory rate, the minute volume and the wasted ventilation.

The beneficial effect of thoracic block during the postoperative period in poor risk children with respiratory disabilities has been reported by Meignier et al (49).

Neuro-endocrine and metabolic effects

The abolition of afferent stimuli transmitted along autonomic as well as sensory pathways may play a major role in the prevention of the endocrine responses to surgery (Table 1). These responses consist of a rise in catecholamine and cortisol levels, negative nitrogen balance, and water and salt retention (50). Some of the results of studies in adults appear to be contradictory and measurements may be influenced by factors such as the type of local anaesthetic used, the presence or absence of adrenaline in the solution, the height and density of the epidural block, and the operative blood loss. However, there is general agreement that, in adults undergoing lower abdominal surgery, epidural anaesthesia extending from T4 to S5 blocks the rise in plasma glucose, cortisol, cyclic AMP and catecholamines (51,52)(Table 2).

Table 1. Effect of epidural anaesthesia on surgically induced changes in endocrine functions. Only the studies marked * were performed in children. Handbook of Epidural Anaesthesia and Analgesia (1985) Covino BG, Scott DB. Schultz Copenhagen.

Endocrine parameters	Surgery	Epidural blockade
Pituitary hormones		
Prolactin	↑	Inhibit
Growth hormone	↑	Inhibit
ACTH *	↑	Inhibit
ADH *	↑	Inhibit
Adrenal and renal hormones		
Cortisol *	↑	Inhibit
Aldosterone	↑	Inhibit
Renin	↑	Inhibit
Epinephrine	↑	Inhibit
Norepinephrine	↑	Inhibit
Pancreatic hormones		
Insulin	-	↓
Glucagon	-	-
Thyroid hormones		
Thyroxine	-	-
Triiodothyronine	↓	-

Table 2. Effect of epidural anaesthesia on surgically induced changes in metabolic functions. Only the studies marked * were performed in children. Handbook of Epidural Anaesthesia and Analgesia (1985) Covino BG, Scott DB. Schultz Copenhagen.

Metabolic parameters	Surgery	Epidural blockade
Glucose *	↑	Inhibit
Lactate	↑	Inhibit
3-hydroxybutyrate	↑	Inhibit
Glycerol	↑	Inhibit
Free fatty acids	↑	Inhibit
Alanine	↓	-
Cyclic AMP	↑	Inhibit

In children under general anaesthesia, even minor lower abdominal surgery is sufficient to produce neuro-endocrine and metabolic responses (Fig. 17.), but caudal block is effective in preventing them (53). However, it has been shown in both adults and children that a block sufficient to provide perfect postoperative analgesia does not suppress the postoperative stress response (54). Lumbar epidural anaesthesia is effective in reducing the cortisol response to peripheral surgical procedures in children (Fig. 18.).

A specific endocrine response has been described which differs in prepubertal boys and adults (55). In the latter, testosterone decreases during surgery under general anaesthesia, but not under epidural anaesthesia. In contrast, testosterone increases significantly during surgery under general anaesthesia in boys. The explanation probably lies in the fact that, in adults, the testes are responsible for 99% of the total testosterone production, whereas in prepubertal boys, the adrenals as well as the testes are involved, and there may also be some peripheral conversion of the precursors of testosterone.

The effects on metabolism of a combination of regional and general anaesthesia have also to be considered. Reinauer and Hollmann (56) found that there was an accumulation of lactic acid associated with the use of halothane. The extent depended on the percentage administered, but the effects were detectable at 0.5%. Since the regional anaesthetic component of the combined technique allows much lighter levels of general anaesthesia to be used, accumulation of lactic acid can be minimised.

Conclusion

The most important differences between children and adults with regard to the physiological effects of central blocks are:

1. The differential action of local anaesthetics on nerve fibres which results in a high success rate for block of the sacral nerve roots.

2. The minimal haemodynamic effects of central blocks in children less than 6 years old which allow the anaesthetist to avoid fluid loading before he administers an epidural or spinal anaesthetic.

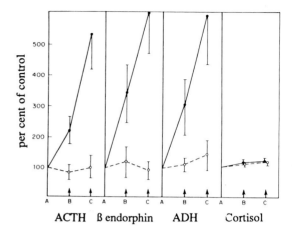

A=Control (induction)
B=3 minutes after induction
C=15 minutes after induction

——— Anaesthesia with Halothane
- - - Caudal block

Fig. 17. Comparison of the endocrine response. E Giaufre (1985) Presse Medicale.

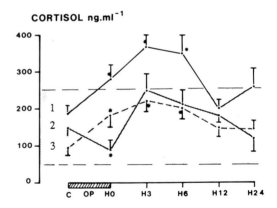

1. Control (n=6)(peripheral surgery)
2. Lumbar epidural (n=7)
3. Thoracic epidural (n=7)

Fig. 18. Changes in the cortisol response (Authors: Murat et al. (54). The dotted lines indicate normal cortisol values in this age group of children, C= pre operative control, HO= end of surgery, H3-H24 post operative hours

References

1. Strichartz G (1985) Interactions of local anesthetics with neuronal sodium channels in: Effects of anesthesia pp 39-52. Covino BG, Fozzard HA, Rehder K, Strichartz G eds American Physiological Society. Bethesda, Maryland.

2. Hille B (1977) Local anesthetics: hydrophilic and hydrophobic pathways for the drug-receptor reaction. J Gen Physiol 69:497

3. Hille B (1977) The pH-dependant rate of action of local anesthetics on the node of Ranvier. J Gen Physiol 69:475

4. Gasser HS, Erlanger J (1929) The role of fibre size in the establishment of a nerve block by pressure or cocaine. Am J Physiol 88:581

5. Nathan PW, Sears TA (1961) Some factors concerned in differential nerve block by local anaesthetics. J Physiol (Lond) 157:565

6. Franz DN, Perry RS (1974) Mechanisms for differential block among single myelinated and non-myelinated axons by procaine. J Physiol (Lond) 236:193

7. Dobbing J (1966) The effect of undernutrition on myelinisation in the Central Nervous System. Biol Neonat 9:132

8. Curless RG (1977) Developmental patterns of peripheral nerve, myoneural junction and muscle: a review. Prog Neurobiol 9:197

9. Blom S, Finnstrom C (1971) Studies on maturity in newborn infants. V.: Motor conduction velocity. Neuropaediatrie 3:129

10. Schulte FJ, Michaelis R, Linke I, Nolte R (1968) Motor nerve conduction velocity in term, preterm and small-for-dates newborn infants. Pediatrics 42:17

11. Wagner AL, Buchthal (1972) Motor and sensory conduction in infancy and childhood: Reappraisal. Develop Med Child Neurol 14:189

12. Covino BG, Scott DB (1985) Handbook of epidural anaesthesia and analgesia. Mechanism of epidural anaesthesia p 36. Schultz Medical Information ApS. Copenhagen, Denmark.

13. Ecoffey C, Dubousset AM, Samii K (1986) Lumbar and thoracic epidural anesthesia for urologic and upper abdominal surgery in infants and children. Anesthesiology 65:87

14. Andrade P (1983) A new interpretation of the origin of extradural space negative pressure. Br J Anaesth 55:85

15. Zarzur E (1984) Genesis of the true negative pressure in the lumbar epidural space. Anaesthesia 39:1101

16. Shah JL (1984) Effects of posture on extradural pressure. Br J Anaesth 56:1373

17. Usubiaga JE, Wilkinski JA, Usubiaga LE (1967) Epidural pressure and its relation to spread of anaesthetic solutions in epidural space. Anesth Analg 46:440

18. Tretjakoff D (1926) Das epidurale Fettgewebe. Z Anat 79:100

19. Galindo A, Hernandez J, Benavides O, Ortegon DE, Munoz S, Bonica JJ (1975) Quality of spinal extradural anaesthesia: the influence of spinal nerve root diameter. Br J Anaesth 47:41

20. Saugbjerg P, Asoh T, Lund C, Kuhl V, Kehlet H (1986) Effects of epidural analgesia on scalp-recorded somatosensory evoked potentials to posterior tibial nerve stimulation. Acta Anaesth Scand 30:400

21. Melzack R, Wall PD (1965) Pain mechanisms: a new theory. Science 150:971

22. Wall PD (1978) The gate control theory of pain mechanisms: a re-examination and re-statement. Brain 101:1

23. Clendinnin HJ, Pehaitis M, Simon EJ (1976) Ontological development of opiate receptors in rodent brain. Brain Res 118:157

24. Simon EJ, Hiller JM (1978) In vitro studies on opiate receptors and their ligands. Fed Proc 37:141

25. Wardlaw SL, Stark R, Barc L, Franz A (1979) Plasma ß-endorphin and B-lipotropin in human fetus at delivery: correlation with arterial pH and P0$_2$. J Clin Endocr Metab 49:888

26. Moss IR, Conner H, Yee WF, Jorio P, Scarpelli EM (1982). Human ß-endorphin-like immunoreactivity (ELI) in the perinatal/neonatal period. J Pediatr 101:443

27. Bonica JJ, Berges PU, Morikawa K (1970) Circulatory effects of peridural block: I-effects of level of analgesia and dose of lidocaine. Anesthesiology 33:619

28. Scott DB, Littlewood DG, Drummond GB, Buckley PF, Covino BG (1977) Modification of the circulatory effects of extradural block combined with general anaesthesia by the addition of adrenaline to lignocaine solutions. Br J Anaesth 49:917

29. Stephen GW, Lees MM, Scott DB (1969) Cardiovascular effects of epidural block combined with general anaesthesia. Br J Anaesth 41:933

30. German PAS, Roberts JG, Prys-Roberts C (1979) The combination of general anaesthesia and epidural block: I-The effects of sequence of induction on hemodynamic variables and blood gas measurements in healthy patients Anaesth Intens Care

7:229

31. Ruston FG (1954) Epidural anaesthesia in infants and children. Can Anaesth Soc J 1:37

32. Fortuna A (1967) Caudal analgesia: a simple and safe technique in paediatric surgery. Br J Anaesth 39:165

33. Arthur DS (1980) Postoperative thoracic epidural analgesia in children. Anaesthesia 35:1131

34. Dohi S, Naito H, Takahashi T (1979) Age-related changes in blood pressure and duration of motor block in spinal anesthesia. Anesthesiology 50:319

35. Murat I, Delleur MM, Esteve C, Egu JF, Raynaud P, Saint-Maurice C (1987) Continuous epidural anaesthesia in children: clinical and haemodynamic implications. Br J Anaesth 59:1441

36. Woods JR, Dandavino A, Murayama K, Brinkman CR, Assali NS (1977) Autonomic control of cardiovascular functions during neonatal development and in adult sheep. Circ Res 40:401

37. Buckley NM, Brazeau P, Gootman PM (1983) Maturation of circulatory responses to adrenergic stimuli. Fed Proc 42:1643

38. Gootman PM, Gootman N, Buckley BJ (1983) Maturation of central autonomic control of the circulation. Fed Proc 42:1648

39. Magrini F (1978) Haemodynamic determinants of the arterial blood pressure rise during growth in conscious puppies. Cardiovasc Res 12:422

40. Wear R, Robinson S, Gregory GA (1982) The effects of halothane on the baroresponse of adult and baby rabbits. Anesthesiology 56:188

41. Seagard JL, Elegbe EO, Hopp FA, Bosnjak ZJ, Von Colditz JH, Kampine JP (1983) Effects of isoflurane on the baroreceptor reflex. Anesthesiology 59:511

42. Wolf WJ, Neal MB, Peterson MD (1986) The hemodynamic and cardiovascular effects of isoflurane and halothane anesthesia in children. Anesthesiology 64:328

43. Arndt JO, Hock A, Stanton-Hicks M, Stuhmeier KM (1985) Peridural anesthesia and the distribution of blood in supine humans. Anesthesiology 63:616

44. Payen D, Ecoffey C, Carli P, Dubousset AM (1987) Pulsed Doppler ascending aortic, carotid, brachial, and femoral artery blood flows during caudal anesthesia in infants. Anesthesiology 67:681

45. McCarthy GS (1976) The effect of thoracic extradural analgesia on pulmonary gas distribution, functional residual capacity and airway closure. Br J Anaesth 48:234

46. Takasaki M, Takahashi T (1980) Respiratory function during cervical and thoracic extradural analgesia in patients with normal lungs. Br J Anaesth 52:1271

47. Murat I, Delleur MM, McGee K, Saint-Maurice C (1985) Changes in ventilatory patterns during halothane anaesthesia in children. Br J Anaesth 57:569

48. Hatch DJ, Hulse MG, Lindahl SGE (1984) Caudal analgesia in children. Influence on ventilatory efficiency during halothane anaesthesia. Anaesthesia 39:873

49. Meignier M, Souron R, Le Neel JC (1983) Postoperative dorsal epidural analgesia in the child with respiratory disabilities. Anesthesiology 59:473

50. Kehlet H (1985) The stress response to anaesthesia and surgery: release mechanisms and modifying factors. Clin Anaesthesiol 2:315

51. Kehlet H, Brandt MR, Prange-Hansen A, Alberti KGMM (1979). Effect of epidural analgesia on metabolic profiles during and after surgery. Br J Surg 66:543

52. Engquist A, Brandt MR, Fernandes A, Kehlet H (1977) The blocking effect of epidural analgesia on the adrenocortical and hyperglycemic responses to surgery. Acta Anaesth Scand 21:330

53. Giaufre E, Conte-Devolx B, Morisson-Lacombe G, Boudouresque F, Grino M, Rousset-Rouviere B, Guillaume V, Oliver C (1985) Anesthesie peridurale par voie caudale chez l´enfant. Etude des variations endocriniennes. Presse Med 14:201

54. Murat I, Walker J, Estève C, Nahoul K, Saint-Maurice C (1988) Effect of lumbar epidural anaesthesia on plasma cortisol levels in children. Can Anaesth SocJ 35:20

55. Boninsegni R, Salerno R, Andreucetti T, Busoni P, Santoro S (1983) Effects of surgery and epidural or general anaesthesia on testosterone, 17-hydroxyprogesterone, and cortisol plasma levels in prepubertal boys. J Steroid Biochem 106:1783

56. Reinauer H und Hollmann S (1966) Der Einfluss der Narkoseart auf den Gehalt an Adeninnucleotiden, Lactat und Pyruvat in Herz, Leber und Milz der Ratte. Anaesthesist 15:327

Pharmacology and pharmacokinetics

Jean Xavier Mazoit and

Anne-Marie Dubousset

Pharmacology and pharmacokinetics of the drugs used in regional anaesthesia

The practice of regional anaesthesia in paediatrics requires knowledge of the physicochemical properties, pharmacokinetics and mechanism of action of the drugs used for such techniques. Differences in anatomy, physiology and metabolism between adults, infants and children may lead to differences in kinetics and dynamics of the drugs. The indications, contra-indications and dosage regimes must therefore be carefully considered if complications are to be avoided.

Glossary of terms

AAG	alpha-1 acid glycoprotein (or orosomucoid). Also called "stress-protein".
AUC	Area under the plasma (or serum) concentration-time curve.
Cl	Total body clearance.
Cl_{int}	Intrinsic clearance, usually intrinsic hepatic clearance. This term represents the maximum ability of the liver to remove a drug from plasma in the theoretical event of liver blood flow being set to infinity.
CNS	Central nervous system
Cmax	Maximum peak plasma concentration
CSF	Cerebrospinal fluid
CVS	Cardiovascular system
HER	Hepatic extraction ratio
pKa	According to the law of mass action, the pKa is the pH at which half of the molecules are in the ionised form and half in the unionised
T1/2or	Half life during the terminal phase.
T1/2z	In the case of prolonged absorption, the terminal half life will be longer after epidural than after intravenous injection.
V or Vz or Vbeta	Volume of distribution calculated according to the slope of the terminal phase.
Vss	Volume of distribution at steady-state. Usually, Vss is smaller than
V Vc	Volume of the central compartment

Fig. 19. Diagram of the structure of the nerve membrane which consists of a lipid bilayer and protein molecules which contain the sodium channels.

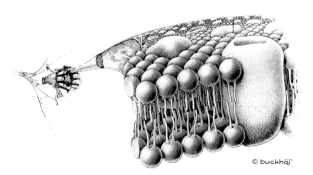

© buckhöj

Local anaesthetics

Structure and physicochemical properties

Structure

Of the two classes of local anaesthetics - esters and amides- the amide group is the one mostly used for paediatric regional anaesthesia. These molecules (Fig 20.) are very similar, with three parts: an aromatic pole responsible for liposolubility, an intermediate chain with the ester or amide link, and a residue responsible for hydrosolubility.

Fig. 20. Structure of local anaesthetic agents

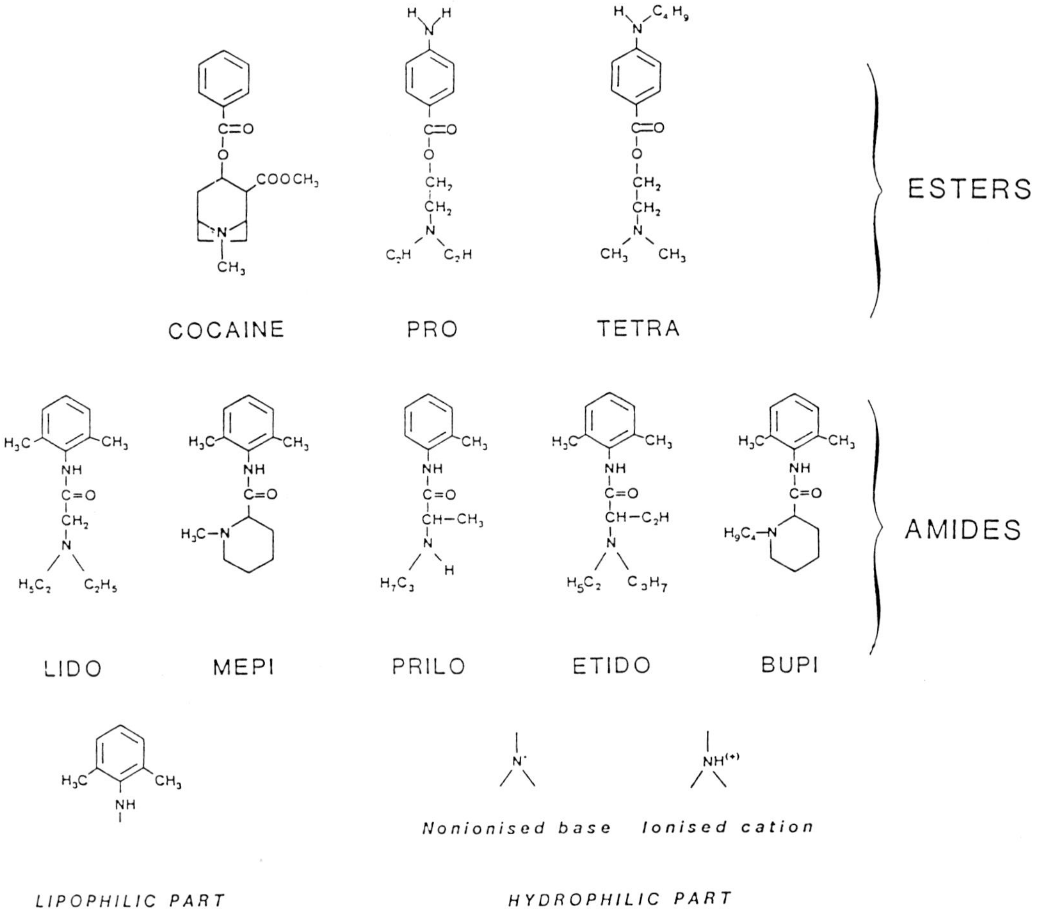

ESTERS

COCAINE   PRO   TETRA

AMIDES

LIDO   MEPI   PRILO   ETIDO   BUPI

Nonionised base   Ionised cation

LIPOPHILIC PART   *HYDROPHILIC PART*

All local anaesthetics are weak bases with a molecular weight between 220 and 288 dalton (Table 1). Three parameters have to be taken into account:

1. pKa
2. liposolubility and molecular weight
3. protein binding

Diffusion in biological fluids depends mainly on ionisation, and therefore on pKa. Diffusion through biological membranes depends mainly on the partition coefficient of the unionised form. Accumulation at and around the site of action is dependent on numerous factors such as protein binding, liposolubility, molecular weight, and association constants with the receptors. However, these latter factors are not so well understood.

pKa and ionisation

The pKa determines the fraction of the drug which is ionised or water soluble, and the fraction which is unionised or membrane soluble. All local anaesthetics are weak bases (Table 3). At pH 7.40, there is 3-4 times more of the ionised fraction available than of the unionised free base. At the average intracellular pH of 6.9, 83% of mepivacaine and 93% of bupivacaine is in the ionised form. Thus, increasing the pKa of a molecule allows it to diffuse better in extracellular fluids. On the other hand, such an increase diminishes its ability to cross membranes.

Table 3. Physicochemical properties of local anaesthetics.

Agent	Molecular Weight (dalton)	pKa (38°C) (1)	Partition Coefficient (3)	Per cent Protein binding	Part Coeff mol-weight binding
Esters					
Procaine	236	8.66	0.02	5.8	0.0010
Chlor- Procaine	271	8.77	0.14		0.0085
Tetracaine	264	8.26	4.10	75.6	0.2500
Amides					
Lidocaine	246	7.55	0.80	77.5	0.0500
Prilocaine	220	7.90	0.90	55.0	0.0600
Etidocaine	(25°C)(2) 276	7.70	141.00	94.0	8.5000
Bupivacaine	(25°C)(2) 288	7.92	27.5	95.6	1.6000

1. Data from Kamaya H, Hayes JJ, Veda I 1983. Dissociation constants of local anesthetics and their temperature dependance. Anesth Analg 62: 1025

2. Data from Tucker GT, Mather LE. 1980. Absorption and disposition of local anesthetics: Pharmacokinetics. In neural blockade in clinical anesthesia and management of pain. Cousins MJ, Brindenbaugh PO, Ed FB Lippicott Co, Philadelphia pp 45
3. N-Heptane/pH 7.4 buffer 25°Celsius

Liposolubility and molecular weight

The aromatic part of the molecule, as well as the length of the lateral chain of the hydrophilic residue, is responsible for liposolubility. According to Fick's law, the more lipophilic a molecule, the better it is able to cross biological membranes. Fenstermacher (1) has demonstrated that the ability of numerous molecules to cross the blood-brain barrier is inversely proportional to their molecular weight. Potency and duration of action seem to be directly related to liposolubility and molecular weight. However, differences in molecular weight between local anaesthetics are not great enough to make an important difference to their effects.

Protein binding

All amide drugs are highly protein bound (Table 1). Potency and duration of action seem to be directly related to protein binding. This may be considered as the result either of 'membrane expansion' or binding to the receptor, or both.

Mechanism of action

Local anaesthetics act by preventing the propagation of the action potential. This inhibition of depolarisation of the axonal membrane is due to the prevention of membrane sodium channels from opening.

The 'modulated receptor hypothesis', advanced almost simultaneously by Hille (2) and by Hondeghem and Katzung (3) in 1977, takes into account most of the features of local anaesthetic actions, especially the anti-arrhythmic effect of lidocaine and the cardiotoxicity of bupivacaine. This theory proposes that local anaesthetics bind more tightly with the sodium channels in the open and inactive states than in the resting state (4).

It has recently been demonstrated that both lidocaine and bupivacaine act as calcium channel blockers (5). Moreover, bupivacaine seems to have a specific action by producing a significant depolarisation of the resting potential. These properties may explain the decrease in the myocardial contractile force as well as the arrhythmias associated with toxic levels of bupivacaine.

Fig. 21. Differential nerve block. The order of blockade is a function of thickness and myelinisation of nerve fibres (AG is Autonomic Ganglion)

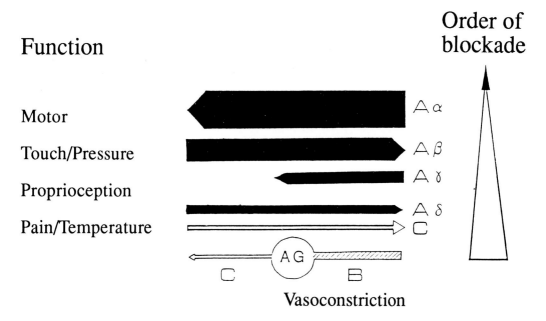

Differential nerve block

The blocking effect of local anaesthetics is considerably influenced by the diameter and degree of myelinisation of nerve fibres. The onset of block and the minimum concentration required for block depend mainly on these two factors, so that thick, heavily myelinated fibres need higher concentrations than thin, unmyelinated ones, and the onset of action is longer for the former (Fig 21). In children, the diameter of the nerve fibres is obviously smaller, and myelinisation less well developed, than in adults. Seemingly in children the diffusion barriers of C fibres are less well developed leading to a wider distribution of analgesia of this quality than in the adult. One clinical consequence of this is that carbonated local anaesthetic solutions, which are sometimes used in adults to shorten the onset time and reduce the risk of failure of a block by improving access to the nerve, are not needed in children.

Frequency-dependent block

Nerve axons are more sensitive to local anaesthetic block when the frequency of impulse traffic is increased. When the impulse frequency is increased on isolated, partially anaesthetised nerve axons, fewer action potentials are conducted. The extent and time-course of frequency-dependent block is partly a function of lipid solubility.

Modulated receptor hypothesis(2,3)

Sodium channels pass into the open and inactive states during depolarisation and local anaesthetics bind more tightly with them when they are in this state. When the channels are in the resting or closed state, the drug unbinds and the channels recover from the block (Fig. 22.).

Two factors are involved in frequency-dependent block:

1. The ease of access of the drug to the receptor - high solubility in membrane lipids is the impotant property governing this.

2. The relative frequency of impulse traffic, and the binding constant affinity or rate-constant for binding.

These factors are important in determining cardiotoxicity. Small molecules with modest lipid solubility, such as lidocaine, bind and unbind very rapidly so that frequency-dependence appears only at high frequency, and these drugs then act as anti-arrhythmics. On the other hand, large molecules with high lipid solubility, such as bupivacaine, dissociate slowly from the channel receptor sites and the frequency-dependence appears at low rates of channel activation. These drugs can therefore act as potent depressors of cardiac conduction. Frequency-dependent block could therefore be a disadvantage in children, because their high heart rates might pre-dispose them to cardiac depression due to local anaesthetics.

Systemic action of local anaesthetics

Local anaesthetics, absorbed from the site of injection and acting systemically, can produce toxic reactions on organs of the body. The fraction available to act on these organs must be viewed in terms of the "free-intermediate model" rather than in terms of the "free-fraction hypo-thesis" (see below).

Fig.22. Various states of the sodium channel. (1) closed. (2) open. (3) inactivated.

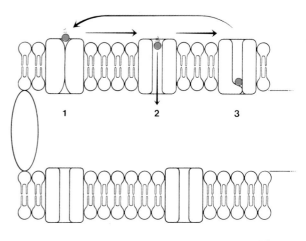

Action on CNS

Amide local anaesthetics cause CNS toxicity, depending upon the dose given. After producing initial drowsiness and an anti-convulsant effect, further increase in dose leads to excitement, convulsions and, finally, depression sufficient to cause coma and respiratory arrest. The first signs of CNS toxicity in awake subjects are light-headedness, and numbness of the tongue and circumoral tissues. Long-acting agents, such as bupivacaine, and short-acting ones, such as lidocaine, do not have the same weight-for-weight toxic potency, bupivacaine being about 3-4 times more toxic than lidocaine. Life support with oxygen, intubation and ventilation are the main measures for the treatment of overdosage. The use of muscle relaxants has been proposed for the treatment of convulsions, but this seems to increase brain uptake of lidocaine (6), and diazepam or even low doses of thiopentone are preferable. The use of succinylcholine should not be necessary if these drugs are effective.

Action on the CVS

Local anaesthetics have "membrane stabilising" properties , which have led to the use of lidocaine as an anti-arrhythmic agent, and to the dreadful cardiovascular accidents observed with the inadvertent intravascular injection of bupivacaine. These effects seem to be due both to direct effects on myocardial fibres and to indirect effects modulated by the CNS (7).

Direct effects

All amide local anaesthetics depress the heart in a dose-dependent manner by causing a decrease in myocardial contractile force, negative bathmotropism, negative dromotropism and negative chronotropism. Heart rate is steadily decreased.

Indirect effects

Reflex activity

Decrease in blood pressure leads to stimulation of the baroreceptor reflex which causes an increase in heart rate.

Central sympathetic stimulation

This is an early sign of CNS toxicity, and leads to an increase in blood pressure, heart rate, cardiac output and myocardial contractile force , all of which are probably mediated by catecholamine release.

In summary, local anaesthetics cause cardiac depression, though this may be masked clinically by reflex and indirect effects. Presumably infants, who have high heart rates, are more prone to the depressant effects compared with adults (4).

Local anaesthetics can also cause cardiac arrhythmias by a central action as demonstrated by the direct application of lidocaine and bupivacaine to the CNS. Heavner (8) and Thomas (9), working almost simultaneously, have shown that introduction of local anaesthetic to the cerebral ventricles of cats (8) and to the medulla of rats (9) induces arrhythmias sometimes severe enough to cause death. On the other hand, intravenous lidocaine has been proposed as a treatment for bupivacaine intoxi-cation (10) on the grounds that lidocaine may displace bupivacaine from the membrane receptors (4). However, the toxicity of both drugs may summate, and further investigations are required to confirm or invalidate this hypo-thesis.

Treatment of CVS toxicity

In cases of massive overdosage due to accidental intravascular injection, several therapeutic measures have been proposed, but life-threatening effects must be treated with oxygenation, tracheal intubation, artificial ventilation, and mild alkalinisation in order to improve the free/bound and the ionised/unionised ratios of the drug. Cardiopulmonary resuscitation should be performed long enough to permit dissociation of the drug from cardiac proteins. It has recently been shown that the intravenous administration of comparatively large doses of adrenaline is a useful therapeutic measure.

Action on the respiratory system

Local anaesthetics seem to have mild to moderate effects upon the respiratory system. It has been shown that systemically available lidocaine has a mild stimulating effect, with an increase in the slope of the ventilatory response to CO_2(11).

Action on metabolism

Methaemoglobinaemia may occur with high doses of prilocaine in adults. Some accidents with low doses in infants have been reported (12) and it seems best to avoid the use of prilocaine in this age group.

Action of additive drugs

Adrenaline is often used in combination with local anaesthetics to delay absorption. Used as a test dose, it may permit detection of an intravascular injection by means of its cardiovascular effects. Its half-life is very short and if it is injected intravascularly, the effects, such as tachycardia (perhaps even associated with dysrhythmia) and vasoconstriction, with hypertension and pallor, are very transient. When adrenaline is used in this way to rule out an intravascular injection, the minimum dose required for recognition of this event is important (13). Halothane anaesthesia, which is often combined with regional anaesthesia in paediatric practice, increases myocardial sensitivity to adrenaline and is theoretically contra-indicated. However, it has been demonstrated that the use of moderate doses,

such as 1ml/kg of a 1:200.000 solution, has no deleterious effect on the heart (14). The influence of atropine is debatable. Secretions are a common problem in paediatric anaesthesia and atropine is given to diminish them, but it causes an increase in heart rate which may make the cardiac response to intravascular adrenaline less obvious. However, the injection in incremental doses is recommended to avoid deleterious effects.

Local disposition

The significance of most of the factors involved in the local disposition of local anaesthetics remains largely unresolved so far as their clinical interest and interrelationship are concerned. However, disposition depends on the volume, force and flow of the injection, diffusion in extracellular fluids and across membranes, and non-specific protein binding. Some studies (15) have shown that systemic disposition (Fig. 23) seems to be enhanced in infants. The concentration needed to produce block is decreased in

Fig. 23. Systemic disposition of local anaesthetic

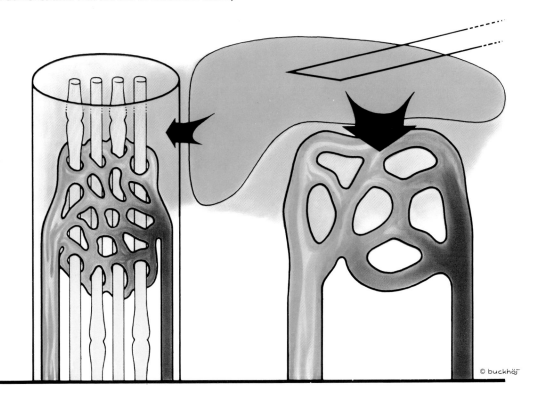

© buckhöj

45

infants and young children, and the addition of adrenaline to bupivacaine results in longer duration of pain relief in children less than 4 years of age compared with older children (16).

Pharmacokinetics

Local diffusion at the site of injection produces the desired effect, which is regional anaesthesia, but diffusion into the blood stream produces concentrations of drug which may possibly result in side effects in the form of toxic reactions (Fig. 24).

The factors which determine blood concentration are not the same after single-shot as after multiple top-up injections. After a single injection, the peak plasma concentration depends mainly upon two factors, the rate of absorption and the volume of distribution. Clearance is of little importance here, whereas during multiple injections or infusions, it is virtually the only factor determining blood concentration in the steady state.

Absorption

It is commonly assumed (17) that the bioavailability of amide drugs injected by routes other than the intravenous is complete. Absorption processes are of major importance in clinical pharmacokinetics and for the prediction of toxic

Fig. 24. Cross-section of the spinal cord and spinal roots. Note that the epidural veins are surrounded by abundant fat.

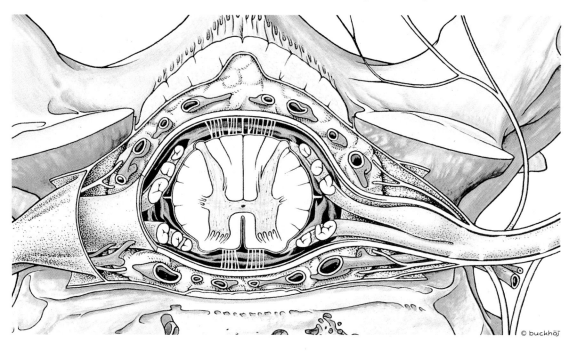

© buckhöj

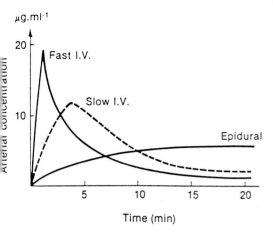

μg.ml⁻¹ (shown as μg.ml·¹ on axis)

Fig. 25. Relationship between arterial concentration of local anaesthetic following rapid I.V., slow I.V., and epidural administration.

reactions. For instance, Tucker and Mather (17) demonstrated that absorption from the epidural space is biphasic. They attributed this to the fact that epidural fat acts as a store in which injected drug can accumulate, and this is responsible for a longer terminal half-life after epidural injection than after intravenous injection. After a single-shot injection, this same process is responsible for the peak plasma concentration being lower than expected. The epidural fat, therefore, has a protective effect against toxic reactions. In infants, the epidural fat is not so abundant as in adults (Fig. 24) so peak plasma concentrations may be expected earlier. Studies by Eyres and colleagues (15) have shown this to be the case.

Speed of injection
Increasing or decreasing the speed of injection has little effect on the rate of absorption of drugs from the epidural space (18). However, an inadvertent intravascular injection may be detected before a serious overdose has been given if the speed of injection is slow enough (Fig. 25).

	Lidocaine	Bupivacaine
Blood/plasma partition coefficient	0.84	0.73
Fraction unbound in plasma	0.36	0.04
Vdss (1/kg)	1.2	0.96
Fraction of drug in body:		
In blood	0.06	0.07
In plasma	0.03	0.04
Unbound in plasma	0.012	0.0018
In extra cellular fluids	0.18	0.23

According to Tozer TN. (1981) Concepts basic to pharmacokinetics. Pharmac Ther 12: 109 with data from ref. 17

Table 4. Distribution of lidocaine and bupivacaine in body (adults)

Disposition
Disposition is dependent on two processes - distribution and elimination - so that terminal half-life is directly proportional to the volume of distribution and inversely proportional to the total body clearance:

$$T\ 1/2 = 0.693 \times \frac{Vd}{Cl}$$

Distribution
Amide local anaesthetics are highly protein bound and extensively distributed outside the blood (Table 4.). At a pH of 7.40, about 3/4 of the local anaesthetic molecules are in the ionised form. On a weight-for-weight basis, the volume of extracellular fluid in the newborn and young infant is about twice that in the adult. The volume of distribution is much larger in infants. As it is known that the protein binding of many drugs is decreased in infancy (19), the blood concentration of the free drug depends on the fraction which is protein- bound, and on the

47

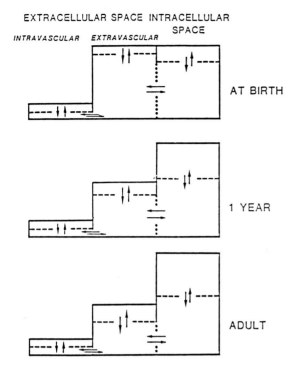

EXTRACELLULAR SPACE INTRACELLULAR SPACE

INTRAVASCULAR   EXTRAVASCULAR

AT BIRTH

1 YEAR

ADULT

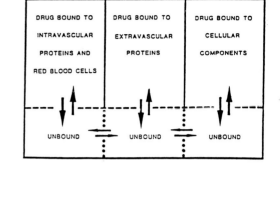

EXTRACELLULAR SPACE   INTRACELLULAR SPACE

INTRAVASCULAR   EXTRAVASCULAR

DRUG BOUND TO	DRUG BOUND TO	DRUG BOUND TO
INTRAVASCULAR	EXTRAVASCULAR	CELLULAR
PROTEINS AND	PROTEINS	COMPONENTS
RED BLOOD CELLS		

UNBOUND   UNBOUND   UNBOUND

Fig. 26 Distribution of local anaesthetics and the relationship between body water compartments and volume of distribution of water soluble drugs. The right panel shows the equibrium process (adapted from Tozer TN. Concepts basic to pharmacokinetics. Pharmac Ther 1981, 12 109-31 with permission). The left panel shows the differences in water repartition in the body according to age, and explains why volume of distribution is expected to be much greater in neonates and young infants than in adults

volume of distribution. One would expect, therefore, that in the steady state, the free drug concentration in blood (in equilibrium with the free drug concentration in extracellular fluids) would be higher in newborn and young infants than in adults (Fig 26).

Lung uptake

It is the arterial concentration of a drug which determines the appearance of toxic reactions. It has been demonstrated that in adults the lung extraction ratio for all amide local anaesthetics is very high (0.8 to 0.9) and as a result there is a considerable difference between mixed venous and arterial concentrations (20). Although the lung thus plays a part in limiting the peak plasma concentrations and slowing the rate of rise to the peak, its role in protecting the patient against toxic reactions is debatable, because the lung is very rapidly saturated.

Elimination

Very little information on pharmacokinetics is available from birth to childhood. A prolongation of the terminal half-life of most drugs has been observed in neonates, but it is impossible to attribute this to the projected increase in the volume of distribution or to a decrease in clearance or to these two factors acting together. Ester and amide local anaesthetics are eliminated after undergoing metabolism (Fig. 27), so that less than 5% is excreted unchanged by the kidney.

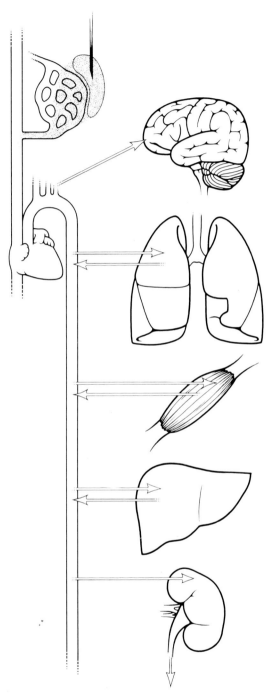

© buckhöj

Fig. 27. Distribution of local anaesthetics in the body

49

Ester metabolism

Metabolism of esters takes place mainly in serum for the commonly used drugs, and plasma hydrolysis by pseudocholinesterases is the major pathway for the metabolism of esters derived from para-amino-benzoic acid (procaine, chloroprocaine and tetracaine). Liver hydrolysis is the predominant pathway for other ester drugs (piperocaine). Further transformations occur before excretion, and the metabolites (especially conjugates with para-amino-benzoic acid) seem to be responsible for the allergic reactions which are sometimes associated with the use of ester local anaesthetics (21). Since these agents share the same metabolic pathway as succinylcholine, it is theoretically possible for prolonged curarisation to result when the two types of drugs are used together (22). In neonates, in vitro studies indicate that the rate of metabolism is decreased compared with adults. The plasma half-life of chloroprocaine in cord plasma has been reported to be twice that of the maternal half-life - 43s as against 21s (23).

Amide metabolism

Amides are metabolised in the liver by oxidative pathways involving cytochrome P450. The drug-metabolising cytochrome P450 level has been found to be almost the same in neonates as in adults (24), so one would expect that the capacity to metabolise amide drugs would also be the same. It seems, however, that this is only true for lidocaine (25). Newborn infants have little capacity for metabolising mepivacaine (26). N dealkylation of bupivacaine cannot occur until several hours after birth (27), but it does seem to take place rather more easily than with mepivacaine. After caudal injection in infants ranging from one to six month of age, bupivacaine clearance exhibited almost the same values as those reported in adults (28). Moreover, all these amide agents have active metabolites. For instance, the N dealkylation of lidocaine to mono-

Fig. 28. Metabolic degradation of lidocaine. Handbook of Epidural Anaesthesia and Analgesia (1985) Covino BG, Scott DB. Schultz Copenhagen.

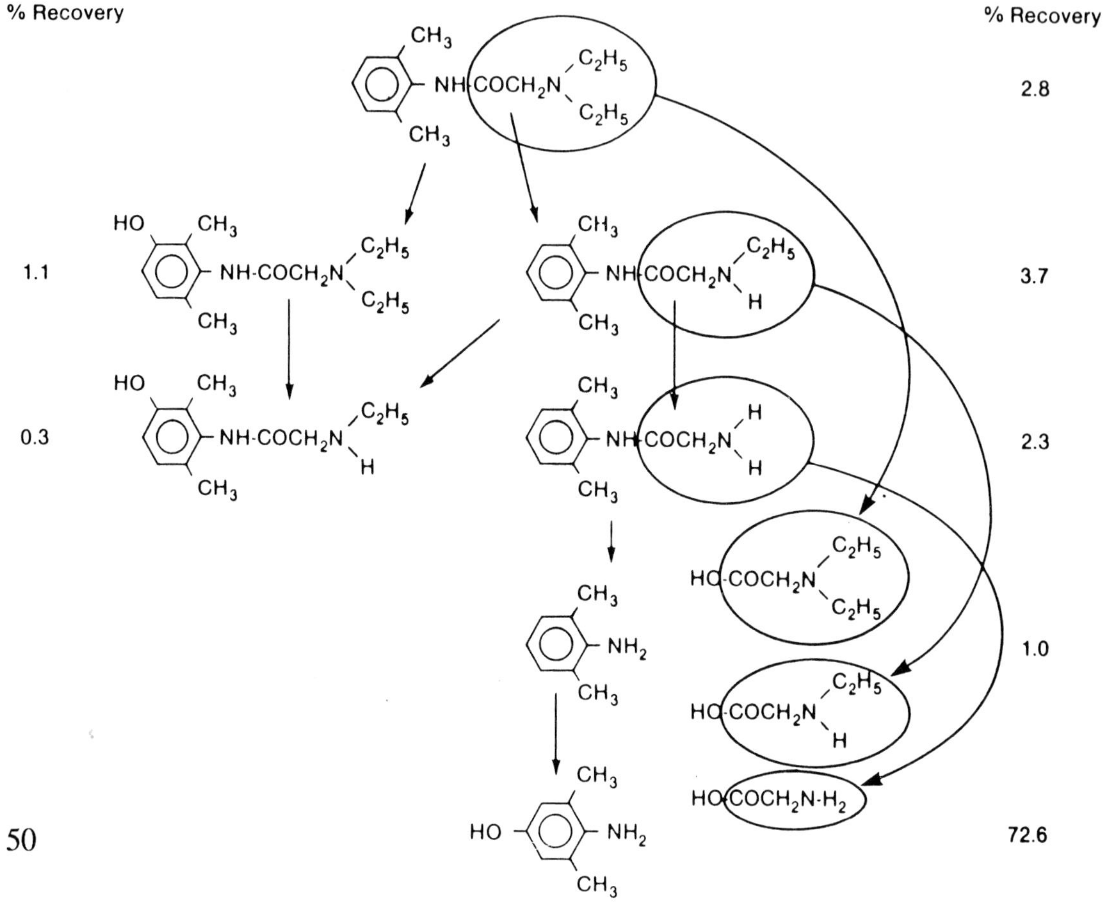

% Recovery

% Recovery

50

ethylglycine xylidine (MEGX) is the major pathway of degradation,(Fig. 28) and MEGX is only slightly less potent and toxic than the parent drug. In neonates, the metabolising capacity for metabolites is the same as in adults. Furthermore, if this capacity decreases, it does so in the same proportion as the metabolising capacity for the parent drug, so that the metabolite/parent drug ratio is the same as in adults.

Hepatic clearance of amide drugs

With the exception of bupivacaine, amide local anaesthetics have relatively high hepatic clearance. Hepatic blood flow is therefore the factor which limits clearance, and the drugs are considered as being "flow-limited". This assumption must be modified in the light of two facts.

Firstly, although lidocaine clearance in neonates is virtually the same as in adults, this is not true for mepivacaine and bupivacaine (see above). Secondly, it has been shown in adults that clearance decreases with time (29). During pro-longed infusion total clearance decreases whereas indocyanine green clearance (reflecting the hepatic blood flow) actually remains unchanged. This fact has been attributed to a product-inhibition by a lidocaine metabolite (29). The same time-dependent decrease in bupivacaine clearance has been shown to occur in the dog (30). Thus, lidocaine and the other agents are at least partially "rate-limited" because the lowering of the intrinsic clearance now becomes the most importance factor.

Table 5. Pharmacokinetics (iv and s.cut) in neonates.

A=Adult, N=Neonate
References
IV in adults: Tucker GT (ref 17)
IV neonates: Mago R, Berlin A, Karlsson K, Kjellmer I. Anesthesia for cesarean section IV: Placental transfer and neonatal elimination of bupivacaine following epidural analgesia for elective cesarean section. Acta Anaesth Scand 20: 141, 1976, and
Brown WU, Bell GC, Lurie AO et al: Newborn blood levels of lidocaine and mepivacaine in the first postnatal day following maternal epidural anesthesia. Anesthesiology 42:698, 1975.
S.cut - Mather LE, Tucker GT (re f 40).

Agent	$T1/2$ (h) A	N	V_z ($1.kg^{-1}$) A	N	Cl ($ml.min^{-1}.kg^{-1}$) A	N	HER A
Lidocaine							
IV	1.6	3	1.2	-	12.7	-	0.63
s.cut	1.8	3.2	1.1	2.8	9.2	10.2	
Mepivacaine							
IV	1.9	9	1.1	-	10.4	-	0.52
s.cut	3.2	8.7	1.0	1.8	5.5	5.2	
Etidocaine							
IV	2.6	-	1.8	-	14.8	-	0.74
s.cut							
Bupivacaine							
IV	3.5	8.1	0.97	-	7.7	-	0.39
s.cut			---			—	

Disposition according to age

The difference in disposition between adults after IV injection and neonates after placental transfer has been studied. Unfortunately, as the dose received after placental transfer is not known, only information on terminal half-life is avail-able (Table 5.). Prolongation of the terminal half-life of lidocaine is compatible with a normal clearance and an increased volume of distribution. The important increase in the terminal half-life of mepivacaine and bupivacaine seems to be due mostly to a decrease in clearance.

Factors affecting disposition

The disposition of a local anaesthetic influences its subsequent pharmacokinetic behaviour and the susceptibility of the organism to it. Many factors affect the disposition. Decrease in body temperature leads to a prolongation in terminal half-life of lidocaine in newborn puppies (31). Low cardiac output decreases splanchnic blood flow- and therefore clearance - in adults (32). Circadian periodicity in CNS susceptibility to lidocaine has been reported in mice (33).

Fig. 29. Protein binding of lidocaine and bupivacaine. This figure simulates the increase in free drug concentration when total concentration increases, according to the following formula

$$Ct = \sum \frac{ni\ Pi\ ki\ cf}{1 + ki\ Cf} + Cf$$

where Ct and Cf are total concentration and free concentration, ni.Pi is the number of sites in the ith class of binding, ki is the dissociation constant for binding of the ith class. The data for lidocaine and bupivacaine binding constants are from Mc Namara PJ et al. Anesth Analg 1981, 60:395, and Coyle DE Anesthesiology 1984, 61:127. Reproduced from Mazoit JX et al. Ann Fr Anesth Réanim 7:,1988 with permission.

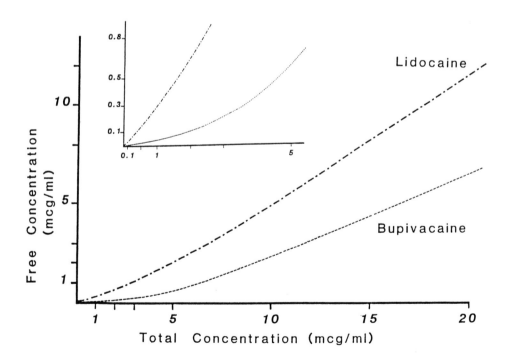

Protein binding

Amide local anaesthetics are extensively bound to proteins in serum (Fig. 29.) and this binding may be expected to provide some protection against toxic reactions (34). The two proteins involved are albumin and alpha-1 acid glycoprotein (AAG), but their binding properties are very different. Albumin has a low affinity for the drug, and virtually never becomes saturated. As a result, the free fraction of a drug increases steadily as the total concentration in the plasma increases. In contrast, AAG has a high affinity for the drug, and a greater number of molecules are bound per mole of albumin. However, it soon becomes saturated and once this saturation threshold is reached, the free fraction of drug increases very rapidly when the total concentration in the plasma increases (Fig 29). Great differences exist between the serum proteins in neonates, young infants and adults. Protein levels are very low at birth and increase in the first months of life to reach adult levels between 6 and 12 months (19). It has been shown that the free fraction of bupivacaine was increased in infants at least until six months of life (28). Moreover, this study showed a negative regression between free fraction and age parallel to the decrease in AAG concentration with age.

Protein binding in relation to organ extraction and toxicity

The "free drug" hypothesis states that only the unbound drug is available for extraction by organs. Until recently, this hypothesis has been accepted without question, despite some contrary evidence such as the high hepatic clearance of some highly bound drugs i.e. propranolol and amide local anaesthetics. Pardridge among others, demonstrated that the circulating drug available for entry into peripheral tissues is not restricted to the free moiety, but includes in part the protein-bound fraction (35). Moreover, great differences in extraction have been demonstrated between organs and between drugs. This "free-inter-mediate" model takes into account the possibility that many factors, such as specific receptors or the presence of free fatty acids at the membrane surface, might be involved in facilitation of the diffusion process.

Protein binding and extraction by individual organs

Central nervous system

Chronic toxicity in adults, in the case of bupivacaine, is clearly related to the free fraction of drug (36). Acute toxicity is not so clearly related, and there are some differences between drugs. Extraction of lidocaine by the rat blood/brain barrier depends on albumin concentration, but is unrelated to AAG concentration (35). Similarly, bupivacaine extraction by the rat brain mainly depends on albumin concentration rather than AAG concentration (37). Thus, the exchangeable bupivacaine in the brain is several times greater than the in vitro unbound fraction.

Liver

There is evidence that the exchangeable local anaesthetic fraction in the liver is several times greater than the free fraction (see hepatic extraction ratio in Table 5). In conclusion, if the concentration of free drug is not the only component of the exchangeable fraction, it appears that it is the free fraction, rather than the total concentration, which determines toxicity. Nevertheless, one must remember that the toxic fraction is several times greater than the free concentration and that differences between acute and chronic toxicity might appear.

Factors influencing protein binding

Serum protein levels and the interaction of the drug with these proteins are the major determinants of the free drug concentration, but acidosis is another important factor and is of interest to the anaesthetist. Both metabolic and respiratory acidosis increase the free fraction of lidocaine and bupivacaine in humans (38, 39). Respiratory acidosis may occur during anaesthesia and it is important to note that it can lead to a sudden increase in the risk of toxicity, even in the absence of repeat, top-up injections. The role of bilirubin is also important, because it discourages the drug from binding with albumin. Neonates suffering from jaundice are therefore highly susceptible to drugs such as the amide local anaesthetics which bind with albumin.

Pharmacokinetics and route of administration

Great differences in pharmacokinetics may be expected to occur from birth through childhood (Table 6). In infancy, the interaction of three factors - more rapid absorption, a larger volume of distribution and lower plasma levels of albumin and AAG - may have wide-ranging effects.

Table 6. Pharmacokinetic parameters of local anaesthetic agents according to the route

AGENT/ROUTE	AGE	DOSE	Cmax (mcg/ml)	tmax (min)	T1/2 (h)	Vss (l/kg)	Cl (ml/kg/ min)	REF.
LIDOCAINE								
Caudal	<1yr	4 mg/kg 1%	2	10-20				Ref 15
	1-10yrs	4 mg/kg 1%	2	10-20				Ref 15
	5yrs	5 mg/kg 1%	2.05	9	2.6	3.05	15.4	Ref 41
	(3.5-7)		(1.6-2.5)	(4-16)	(1.25-6.2)	(2.01-5.29)	(9.8-21.2)	
	2.6yrs	11 mg/kg 1.5%	2.20	30-45				1
	±0.5 SEM	Epineph 1/200.000						
	Adults	6 mg/kg 2%	2.47-0.23	45				2
	40yrs	Epineph 1/200.000	(50)					
Lumbar	Adults	300-400 mg 2%	2.3	24	2.33	2.5	11.65	3
MEPIVACAINE								
Caudal	3.3yrs	11 mg/kg 1.5%	2.53	45				1
	±0.6 SEM	Epineph. 1/200.000						
BUPIVACAINE								
Caudal	<1yr	3 mg/kg 0.25%	1.4	15-20	Corresponding arterial data:			4
	>1yr	3 mg/kg 0.25%	1.27	20-30	Cmax: 1.6 mcg/ml - Tmax 15-20 min			
	1-6 months	2.5 mg/k g 0.25%	0.97	28	7.7	3.9	7.1	Ref 28
	7.25	2.5 mg/kg 0.25%	1.25	29	4.6	2.7	10	Ref 42
	(5.5-10)		(0.95-1.64)	20-40	(2.9-5.3)	(1.6-3.3)	(8.3-11.7)	
	2.4+0.7	3.7 mg/kg 0.5%	0.7	30-45				1
	(SEM)	Epineph 1/200.000						
	Adults	2.2 mg/kg 0.75%	0.86±0.22	30				2
	40yrs	Epineph 1/200.000	(SD)					
Lumbar	3-36months	3.25 mg/kg 0.5%	1.35+0.17	20				Ref 43
		Epineph 1/200.000						
	1.5-11yrs	1.7 mg/kg 0.25%	0.64	19	3.8	3.4	11.0	5
		Epineph 1/200.000						
	(SEM)	20						
	Adults	150 mg 0.5%	1.14		2.8			6
		Epineph 1/200.000						
Axillary Plexus	Adults	3 mg/kg 0.5%	1.44	15-30				7
			(0.68-3.33)					
Intercostal	55±11months	3 mg/kg 0.5%	1.4±1.210	2.27			Ref 44	
		Epineph 1/200.000						

1. Takasaki et al (1984) Anesth Anal 66:337
2. Freund et al (1984) Anesth Anal 63:1017
3. Inoue et al (1985) Anesthesiology 63:304
4. Eyres et al (1983) Anesth Intens Care 11:20
5. Murat et al (1988) Eur J Anaesth 5:113
6. Wilkinson et al (1970) Anesthesiology 63:304
7. Tuominen et al (1983) Acta Anaesth Scand 27:303

Topical anaesthesia of the airway

After topical anaesthesia of the airway, the peak plasma concentration of lidocaine occurs very early in patients younger than 3 years of age (15). Concentrations higher than 8mcg.ml^{-1} have been observed after the application of 4mg.kg^{-1} of 4% lidocaine, and the concentration/time curves resemble the intravenous pattern. Care must be taken in infants and young children because the greater part of the dose is absorbed almost immediately by this route.

Subcutaneous injection

After subcutaneous injection in neonates, it has been shown that the manner in which the terminal half-life of local anaesthetics is prolonged varies according to the drug used (Table 5 p. 51). The extent of metabolism of lidocaine, assessed as total body clearance, is the same in neonates and adults (40). The observed prolongation of the half-life is due to the greater volume of distribution. On the other hand, a marked decrease in the clearance of mepivacaine has been observed (40). Clearance of bupivacaine is also decreased, but one would not expect this to be so important, and the drug seems to be safe in this age group if multiple injections and top-ups are avoided.

Epidural anaesthesia

Caudal epidural anaesthesia

After caudal epidural anaesthesia in children, blood levels of both lidocaine and bupivacaine, given on a weight basis, are very similar to adults, and this is true even for young infants (Table 6). Again, maximum peak concentrations and the time taken to reach the peak are similar to the figures obtained after caudal or lumbar epidural block in adults. It is important to remember that arterial concentrations are slightly higher and appear slightly earlier than mixed venous ones. On the other hand, there are, not surprisingly, differences in disposition. Ecoffey and colleagues (41,42) found an increased total body clearance of both lidocaine and bupivacaine in children between 4 and 10 years compared with adult data, whereas Mazoit and colleagues

(28) found a bupivacaine clearance in infants between 1 and 6 months similar to the adult values. In this latter study the free fraction was found to be markedly increased in young infants. Caution must therefore be exercised in the use of bupivacaine in infants of less than 6 months of age.

Low thoracic or high lumbar epidural anaesthesia

After low thoracic or high lumbar epidural anaesthesia in infants between 3 and 36 months, blood concentrations of bupivacaine (with adrenaline, and given on a weight basis) are also below toxic levels (43).

Blood levels after other routes of administration

After intercostal block, rapid absorption has been observed both in children and adults (44)(Table 6). Although the concentrations observed were just below toxic levels, care should be taken (as in adults) when this technique is used in children. No data are as yet available for other routes.

Effect of added adrenaline

The effect of adding adrenaline (usually 1:200.000) to both lidocaine and bupivacaine is to decrease the maximum concentration and delay absorption. It is of interest that this occurs to a greater extent than is usually observed in adults, especially with bupivacaine (Table 6). In addition to the kinetic effects, this can lead to prolonged duration of pain relief, especially in children under 4 years of age (16).

In summary, blood levels in children - even in infants - after different routes of administration are very similar to those observed in adults. Nevertheless, care should be taken because no data are as yet available regarding the free drug concentration.

Drug interactions

Drug interactions may possibly occur with local anaesthetics themselves, with drugs used for premedication or concurrent general anaesthesia, or with other drugs used for long term therapy (Table 7).

Mixtures of local anaesthetics

These are commonly used in clinical practice, though their efficiency is debatable from the clinical point of view (45) and it is certainly offset by a proven increase in toxicity (46). Interactions which involve displacement of a local anaesthetic from its binding site lead to an increased free fraction in the serum.
Unless precise data for a specific mixture is available, it is best to calculate the toxic dose of a mixture as if it were made up entirely of the most toxic drug.

Interactions with drugs used in premedication and general anaesthesia

No interaction involving protein binding has been reported between local anaesthetics and drugs used for premedication or for concurrent general anaesthesia (Table 7). On the other hand, volatile anaesthetics (47) have been claimed to offer a protective effect against toxic reactions involving the CNS, though it is not clear whether this is true protection or whether adverse reactions due to excessive concentrations of local anaesthetic are merely concealed by general anaesthesia. Although no precise data are available, the use of enflurane in concentrations in excess of 2.5%, together with local anaesthetics, may theoretically be hazardous. However, no adverse reactions have been reported in infants and children when complementary light general anaesthesia was used (48).

Interac. drug	Mechanism	clin. sign.
Cimetidine	oxidative pathway	+++
	hepatic blood flow	(expected)
Propranolol	id	++
Calcium channel	direct interaction	++++
blockers		(dangerous)
	Binding protein involved:	
Diazepam	Albumin	0
Etidocaine	AAG/Albumin	?
Free fatty acids	AAG/Albumin	0
Lidocaine	AAG/Albumin	?
Mepivacaine	AAG	++
Pethidine	Albumin	0
Progesterone	AAG	0
Thiopental	Albumin	0

Table 7. Interactions between bupivacaine and adjuvant drugs adapted from Denson DD ref 46

Interactions with other medications

Little information is at present available on the interaction of local anaesthetics and other highly protein-bound drugs. Of the latter, phenytoin is commonly used in paediatric practice and, in the absence of data, it is questionable whether regional anaesthesia should be performed in patients receiving this therapy. Increased cardiovascular toxicity of calcium channel blockers has been described when regional anaesthesia had been used (49). This increased toxicity is caused both by the direct additive effects of the drugs and by the presence of sympathetic block. The use of local anaesthetics must therefore be avoided in patients receiving such therapy. Drugs such as cimetidine and propranolol which decrease oxidative pathways and/or hepatic blood flow would be expected to decrease the clearance of local anaesthetics, and this has in fact been shown to occur with propranolol (50). In conclusion, relatively few interactions have yet been reported between local anaesthetics and other drugs, but of those known to exist, the interaction with calcium channel blockers is the most dangerous.

Opioids

Narcotics

Structure and mechanism of action

The use of narcotics in paediatric regional anaesthesia is usually restricted to epidural analgesia in which they may be given alone or mixed with local anaesthetics. The structure of narcotics is not so specific as that of local anaesthetic drugs. However, all these molecules have a similar pKa and all are more or less lipophilic. Morphine is only slightly lipophilic, with a partition coefficient close to that of lidocaine (1.4), while other drugs such as fentanyl have very strong lipophilicity (part. coeff.=813). They are believed to act by stimulating inhibitory descending pathways in the dorsal horn region of the spinal cord (51). They produce prolonged pain relief. This analgesia is insufficient for surgical procedures but provides excel-lent postoperative analgesia, and the possibility of using epidural opioids in the treatment of chronic pain is an area of great interest. Epidural opioids produce hardly any cardiovascular effects, but they may cause side effects. The main problem is respiratory depression.

Respiratory depression

Early and late respiratory depression may occur both with morphine and fentanyl (51). It is very uncommon in patients previously made tolerant to opioids, and there have been no reports to date in patients treated for chronic pain. Early depression seems to be due to the systemically absorbed drug, while late depression may be caused by transport to the brain by the vertebral venous plexus rather than by the CSF (51). However, children have the same potential for respiratory depression as adults (52). Respiratory depression may be antagonised by naloxone, but a prolonged infusion (10mcg/kg/h) must be used.

Other side effects

These include nausea and vomiting, urinary retention and, exceptionally, pruritus. Urinary retention may be treated with IV naloxone. These side effects are comparatively common (53) and may place a limit on the usefulness of epidural narcotics in clinical practice.

Pharmacokinetics

After epidural morphine, systemic absorption is rapid, with a t max occuring at 10.3 min (53). The maximum plasma concentration is usually far below that required to produce respiratory depression, and elimination occurs at the same rate as after IV injection (53).

Clinical implications

Local anaesthetics, despite a low therapeutic index, and narcotics, despite the risk of respiratory depression, seem to be safe at these dosages.

The most important clinical implications arising from a study of the pharmacokinetics of drugs used in regional anaesthesia are as follows:
1. The predicted decrease in protein binding of local anaesthetics in infants may lead to toxic reactions, especially if accidental intravascular injection occurs.
2. Acidosis leads to displacement of local anaesthetics from the serum proteins and, therefore, to an increased risk of toxicity.
3. Regarding mixtures of local anaesthetics, precise data is rarely available, so it is wise to calculate the dose of a mixture as if the total dose to be injected were made up of the most toxic drug.
4. The combined effects of local anaesthetics and calcium channel blockers may lead to profound cardiac depression.
5. Adrenaline, used as a test for intravascular injection, does not have the same diagnostic value in infants and young children as in adults. Tachycardia may be very transient. Profound pallor, hypertension and arrhythmias, if they occur, are the important signs.

References

1. Fenstermacher JD, Rapoport SI (1984) The blood-brain barrier. In Handbook of physiology, The microcirculation, ed. by EM Renkin, CC Michel, Washington DC, American Physiological Society 969
2. Hille B (1977) Local anesthetics: Hydrophilic and hydrophobic pathways for the drug-receptor reaction. J Gen Physiol 69:497
3. Hondeghem LM, Katzung BG (1977) Time-and voltage dependant interactions of antiarrhythmic drugs with cardiac sodium channels. Biochem Biophys Acta 472:373
4. Clarkson CW, Hondeghem LM (1985) Evidence for a specific receptor site for lidocaine, quinidine

and bupivacaine associated with cardiac sodium channels in guinea pig ventricular myocardium. Cir Research 56:496

5. Coyle DE, Sperelakis N (1987) Bupivacaine and lidocaine blockade of calcium-mediated slow action potentials in guinea-pig ventricular muscle. J Exp Pharmacol Ther 242:1001

6. Simon RP, Benowitz NL, Culala S (1984) Motor paralysis increases brain uptake of lidocaine during status epilepticus. Neurology 34:384

7. Edouard A, Berdeaux A, Langloys J, Samii K, Giudicelli JF, Noviant Y (1986) Effects of lidocaine on myocardial contractility and baroreflex control of heart rate in conscious dogs. Anesthesiology 64:316-321

8. Heavner JE (1986) Cardiac dysrhythmias induced by infusion of local anesthetics into the lateral cerebral ventricle of cats. Anesth Analg 65:133

9. Thomas RD, Behbehami MM, Coyle DE, Denson DD (1986) Cardiovascular Toxicity of Local Anesthetics: an Alternative Hypothesis. Anesth Analg 65:444

10. Davis NL, de Jong RH (1982) Successful resuscitation following massive bupivacaine overdose. Anesth Analg 61:62

11. Labaille T, Clergue F, Samii K, Ecoffey C, Berdeaux A (1985) Ventilatory response to CO2 following intravenous and epidural lidocaine. Anesthesiology 63:179

12. Duncan PG, Kobrinski N (1983) Prilocaine-induced methemoglobinemia in a Newborn Infant. Anesthesiology 59:75

13. Moore DC, Batra MS (1981) The components of an effective test dose prior to epidural block. Anesthesiology 55:693

14. Maze M, Denson DM Jr. (1983) Aetiology and treatment of halothane induced arrythmias. Clinics in Anaesthesiology 1:301

15. Eyres RL, Kidd J, Oppenheim R, Brown TCK (1978) Local Anaesthetic plasma levels in children. Anesth Intens Care 6:243

16. Warner MA, Kundel SE, Offord KO, Atchison SR, Dawson B (1987) The effects of Age, Epinephrine, and Operative Site on Duration of Caudal Analgesia in Pediatric Patients. Anesth Anal 66:995

17. Tucker GT (1986) Pharmacokinetics of local anaesthetic agents. Br J Anaesth 58:717

18. Scott DB, Jebson PJR, Boyes RN (1973) Pharmacokinetic study of the local anaesthetics bupivacaine and etidocaine in man. Br J Anaesth 45:1010

19. Morselli Pl, Franco-Morselli R, Borsi L (1980) Clinical pharmacokinetics in newborns and infants. Age-related differences and therapeutic implications. Clin Pharmacokin 5:485

20. Jorfeldt L, Levois DH, Lofstrom JB, Post C (1979) Lung uptake of lidocaine in healthy volunteers. Acta Anaesth Scand 23:567

21. Covino BM, Vassalo (1976) Local anesthetics. Mechanism of action and clinical use.p 114. Grune and Stratton, New York

22. Salgado AS (1968) The distribution of procaine in human blood: relation to potentiation of succinylcholine. Anesthesiology 29:1040

23. Finster M, Perel JM, Hinswarko N et al (1974) Pharmacodynamics of 2-chloroprocaine (nesacaine), an ester type local anesthetic. Fourth Europ Cong Anesth Amsterdam. Excerpta Medica 330:189

24. Rane A, Sjoqvist F, Orrenius S (1971) Cytochrome P-450 in human fetal liver microsomes. Chem Biol Interactions 3:305

25. Blankenbaker WL, Di Fazio CA, Berry FA (1975) Lidocaine and its metabolites in the newborn. Anesthesiology 42:325

26. Brown WU, Bell GC, Lurie AO et al (1975) Newborn blood levels of lidocaine and mepivacaine in the first postnatal day following maternal epidural anesthesia. Anesthesiology 42:698

27. Di Fazio CA (1979) Metabolism of local anaesthetics in the foetus, newborn and adult. Br J Anaesth 51:29

28. Mazoit JX, Denson DD, Samii K (1988) Pharmacokinetics of Bupivacaine following Caudal Anesthesia in Infants. Anesthesiology 68:387

29. Bax NDS, Tucker GT, Woods HF (1980) Lignocaine and indocyanine green kinetics in patients following myocardial infarction. Br J Clin Pharmacol 10:353

30. Mazoit JX, Lambert C, Berdeause A, Gerard JL, Froideveause R (1988) Pharmacokinetics of bupivacaine after short and prolonged infusions in conscious dogs. Anesth Anal 67:961-6

31. Morishima Ho, Mueller-Henbach E, Shnider SM. 1971. Body temperature and disappearance of lidocaine in newborn puppies. Anesth Analg 50:938

32. Feely J, Wade D, Mc Allister CB, Wilkinson GR, Robertson D (1982) Effect of hypotension on liver blood flow and lidocaine disposition. N Engl J Med 14:866

33. Lutsch EF, Morris RW (1967) Circadian periodicity in susceptibility to lidocaine hydrochloride. Science 156:100

34. Tucker GT, Mather LE (1979) Clinical

pharmacokinetics of local anesthetics. Clin Pharmacokinet 4:241

35. Pardridge WM, Sakiyama R, Fierer G (1983) Transport of propanolol and lidocaine through the rat blood-brain barrier. J Clin Invest 71:900

36. Denson DD, Myers JA, Hartrick CT, Pither CP, Coyle DE, Raj PP (1984) The relationship between free bupivacaine concentration and central nervous system toxicity. Anesthesiology 61:A211

37. Terasaki T, Pardridge WM, Denson DD (1986) Differential effect of plasma protein binding of bupivacaine on its in vivo transfer into the brain and salivary glands of rats. J Pharmacol Exp Ther 239:724

38. Mc Namara PJ, Slaughter RL, Pieper JA, Wyman MG, Lalka D (1981) Factors influencing serum protein binding of lidocaine in humans. Anesth Analg 60:395

39. Denson DD, Coyle D, Thompson G, Myers J (1984) Alpha 1-acid glycoprotein and albumin in human serum bupivacaine binding. Clin Pharmacol Ther 35:409

40. Mather LE, Tucker GT (1978) Pharmacokinetics and biotransformation of local anesthetics. Int Anesthesiol Clin 16:23

41. Ecoffey C, Desparmet J, Berdeaux A, Maury M, Giudicelli JF, Saint-Maurice C (1984) Pharmacokinetics of lignocaine in children following caudal anaesthesia. Br J Anaesth 56:1399

42. Ecoffey C, Desparmet J, Berdeaux A, Maury M, Giudicelli JF, Saint Maurice C (1985) Bupivacaine in children: pharmacokinetics following caudal anesthesia. Anesthesiology 63:447

43. Ecoffey C, Dubousset AM, Samii K (1986) Lumbar and thoracic epidural anesthesia for urologic and upper adbominal surgery in infants and children. Anesthesiology 65:87

44. Rothstein P, Arthur GR, Feldman HS, Kopf GS, Covino BG (1986) Bupivacaine for intercostal nerve blocks in children: blood concentrations and pharmacokinetics. Anesth Anal 65:625

45. Seow LT, Lips FJ, Cousins MJ, Mather LE (1982) Lidocaine and bupivacaine mixtures for epidural blockade. Anesthesiology 56:177

46. Denson DD (1985) Recent advances in clinical pharmacology of local anesthetics. Proceedings of the fourth MAPAR-Bicêtre. Ed by MAPAR-Bicêtre 161

47. Yoshikawa K, Mima T, Egawa T (1968) Blood level of Marcain (LAC-43) in axillary plexus blocks, intercostal nerve blocks and epidural anaesthesia. Acta Anaesth Scand 12:1

48. Schulte Steinberg O (1988) Neural blockade for pediatric surgery. In neural blockade in clinical anesthesia and management of pain. Cousins MJ, Bridenbaugh PO, Ed. FB Lippincott CO, Philadelphia, p. 672

49. Edouard A, Froideveaux R, Berdeaux A, Ahmad R, Samii K, Noviant Y (1987) Bupivacaine accentuates the cardiovascular depressant effects of verapamil in conscious dogs. Eur J Anaesth 4:249

50. Bax NDS, Tucker GT, Lennard MS, Woods HF (1985) The impairment of lignocaine clearance by propranolol-major contribution from enzyme inhibition. Br J Clin Pharmac 19:597

51. Cousins MJ, Mather LE (1984) Intrathecal and epidural administration of opioids. Anesthesiology 61:276

52. Attia J, Ecoffey C, Sandouk P, Gross JB, Samii K (1986) Epidural Morphine in Children: Pharmacokinetics and CO_2 sensitivity. Anesthesiology 65:87

53. Glenski JA, Warner MA, Dawson B, Kaufman B (1984) Postoperative use of epidurally administered morphine in children and adolescents. Mayo Clin Proc 59:530

Psychological aspects

Elisabeth Giaufré

"Although surgical procedures are necessary for the life and health of a patient, they can produce acute anxiety. The adult recovers quite quickly from the emotional stress of surgery and he is not necessarily affected by it afterwards, but it is different for a child" (1).

Factors independent of anaesthesia (2)

Age and separation from the parents

Schaffer and Callender (3) have shown that hospitalisation and separation from the parents has little effect on children up to the age of 7 months. Thereafter, a child becomes increasingly aware of its surroundings, so that by the age of three, major problems can occur. It has even been suggested (4) that, where possible, elective surgery should be deferred in this age group. By the age of 6, a child has developed a degree of independence and he is more likely to understand the need for surgery. He can also express his anxiety, so it is easier to re-assure him.

Time in the hospital (5)

The shorter the time a child spends in hospital, the better. A young child's initial response to parental separation is one of obvious distress. As time passes, the child becomes quieter and it is tempting to assume that he has "settled in" and has adjusted to his new environment. This apparent tranquility is deceptive, and psychiatrists have shown that, in children subjected to prolonged hospitalisation, it represents not a calm acceptance of separation, but despair. Such children often show regressive behaviour when they return home.

Personality and previous surgical experience

Children, like adults, vary greatly in their personality and their attitude to surgery (6). Sensible and factual preparation by the parents is helpful, and honesty is essential. Previous hospital experiences naturally affect a child's attitude, so it is important that his first admission should be as pain-free and atraumatic as possible. If the first experience was distressing, the causes must be elicited and every effort made to avoid or minimise them during the present admission. This may not be easy if the child has been admitted for further surgery and may again suffer from unpleasant side-effects such as blood loss and vomiting. In this context, it is perhaps significant that adenoidectomy is the operation most frequently remembered by children.

False information

If a child is unduly anxious when he comes into hospital for the first time, it is usually because he has been alarmed by information obtained from a variety of sources. Medical matters are often dealt with on television in an over-dramatised fashion and do little to re-assure. Older children occasionally take pleasure in talking about injections, facemasks, blood and wounds. Parents may unintentionally do harm by concealing the true purpose of the visit to hospital or by imparting inaccurate information.

Sex

The sex of a child has no significant influence on its psychological reaction to hospitalisation or surgery (7).

Factors dependent on anaesthesia

Pre-operative visit
The anaesthetist who intends to perform regional anaesthesia in children should first gain experience in its use in adults. He should also be experienced in paediatric general anaesthesia and in the management of children. It is easier to explain things to a child who knows little or nothing than to re-assure him after he has picked up alarming or misleading information, so it is best if the anaesthetist visits the child the same day as the surgeon. The object of the visit is to explain regional anaesthesia to the child and its parents and to obtain their consent. This presents no difficulty for the experienced anaesthetist if regional anaesthesia is indeed the best choice for the child.

Child

Regional anaesthesia with general anaesthesia
If the two techniques are to be combined, the child should be psychologically prepared as for general anaesthesia (8). However, if regional analgesia is to be continued into the post-operative period, honest explanations are needed so that the child is prepared for any numbness, paraesthesiae or motor weakness which may occur. It should be pointed out to him that these mild side-effects are a small price to pay for his post-operative comfort.

Regional anaesthesia alone
When describing the technique to the child, it is important to avoid the use of frightening words such as "needles" and "injections". The method of testing the block before surgery should be outlined, and it should be emphasised that there will be no pain during and after surgery; indeed, he can be encouraged to sleep during the procedure. The likely duration of the block and the sensations to be expected when it begins to wear off should be mentioned.

Children who have received successful regional anaesthesia a few days previously are valuable allies and they often give the best explanations. An apprehensive child is more likely to be re-assured by a fellow patient than by a doctor.

Parents
A mother who has had an epidural block for delivery can also give re-assurance and, because she has first-hand knowledge of regional anaesthesia, it will not be difficult to convince her of the benefits for her child. Parents who have no such knowledge require more detailed explanations, and simple diagrams (shown out of sight of the child) are useful for illustrating the different techniques, particularly spinals and epidurals.

The amount of information expected by parents and given by anaesthetists varies widely between different countries and cultures and even between different centres in the same country. The disadvantages and possible complications of a technique must be discussed with the parents with due regard for the prevailing climate of medicolegal opinion.

Parents frequently express anxiety about the dangers of regional anaesthesia, particularly the risk of permanent paralysis. They may also be anxious about their child being conscious during surgery and they may require guidance about their role in the child's management after surgery. They often have questions about the prevention of post-operative pain, and if a continuous block is to be used, the technique should be discussed and the advantages emphasised.

At the end of the anaesthetist's visit, the parents should be able to understand the reasons why regional anaesthesia has been chosen, and they should be convinced that it is a reasonable choice. The child too should benefit from the re-assurance that comes with understanding, and he should be unafraid of the procedure.

Staff
It is particularly important that the staff should be accustomed to looking after children in the anaesthetic room and operating theatre, because the requirements of children differ from those of adults. For example, the presence of parents in the anaesthetic room should be encouraged whenever possible, not resisted; fruit flavours in the facemask may be used to make an inhalation induction more pleasant; items of anaesthetic equipment can often be made colourful, attractive and even humorous; preparation of equipment must take place out of sight of the child; and the staff must be expert in getting their own way without resorting to force. If an intravenous

infusion is required, it should be set up at the time of induction, before the block. With regard to the search for paraesthesias in peripheral nerve blocks, it should be stressed that constant questioning for the occurrence of paraesthesias by the staff, although well-intentioned, ought to be avoided and left solely to the anaesthetist performing the procedure.

If the child is to be operated on under regional anaesthesia alone, additional factors become important. The method of testing the block must be effective, but testing should not be started before analgesia can reasonably be expected. Particular care must be taken to ensure that no painful stimulus is accidentally applied to an unanaesthetised part of the body. If the child is sedated, sudden noise must be avoided and the atmosphere in the operating theatre must be calm, because the sense of hearing is often retained after other senses have been obtunded. All staff must keep in mind that the child is under regional anaesthesia.When the block is being performed and during the operation itself, the anaesthetist or a nurse well known to the child should talk to him, either re-inforcing previous explanations or distracting his attention, whichever is appropriate.

When the child returns to the ward, the nurses should be aware that he has received regional anaesthesia and should be ready to re-assure him if he is unable to feel his legs, and again if he becomes anxious as sensation returns to normal. Undesirable side-effects can be minimised if high concentrations of local anaesthetic drug are avoided so that motor block does not occur with caudals and epidurals. Alternatively, specific blocks, such as penile block, may be used.

Summary

Throughout this book, many advantages are claimed for regional anaesthesia in children. Post-operative pain prevention (10) is one of the most important because, if regional techniques are performed skillfully and with careful pre-operative explanation, they can do much to minimise the adverse psychological effects of surgery.

References

1. Pearson G (1941) Effect of operative procedures on the emotional life of the child. Am J Dis Child 62
2. Kay B (1977) Psychological effects of anaesthesia in children. Acta Anaesth Belg 28
3. Shaffer HR, Callender WM (1959) Psychological effects of hospitalisation in infancy. Pediatrics 24:528
4. Hodges R (1960) Induction of anaesthesia in young children. Lancet 82
5. Hain WR (1980) Children in hospital. Anaesth 35:949
6. Benson F, Reinard T (1960) Mental side reactions in paediatric anaesthesia. Acta Anaesth Scand 4:199
7. Vernon D, Shulman J, Foley J (1966) Changes in children's behaviour following hospitalisation. Amer J Dis Child 111:581
8. Kay B (1981) Children and anaesthesia. Anaesth 36:326
9. Kenneth F (1975) Regional anaesthesia for infants and children. Intern Anaesth clinics 13:19
10. Andre V (1988) L'anesthésie peridurale vue par le pediatre et l'enfant. Médical Doctor Graduate Thesis. Marseille

General aspects of management

Ottheinz Schulte Steinberg and

Isabelle Murat

Introduction

Paediatric anaesthetists have traditionally been unenthusiastic about regional anaesthesia. They have been influenced by the belief that children have a basic fear of the unknown, such as the operating room and the strangely dressed people they meet there, and a strong dislike of all medical procedures and instruments, particularly injections and needles. In addition, paediatric anaesthetists have, in the past, frequently lacked experience in regional blocks, and surgeons have been ignorant of their advantages compared with general anaesthesia. It used to be assumed that the combination of regional with general anaesthesia carried with it the risks of both. It is now recognised that the opposite is true. Regional anaesthesia does help to avoid some of the complications of general anaesthesia and it is more accurate to say that the combination of the two techniques carries with it the benefits of both. For example, in the case of circumcision, a regional block avoids laryngospasm and cardiac responses to pain as well as the need for high concentrations of halothane and the accumulation of lactic acid which this causes. On the other hand, general anaesthesia tends to prevent toxic reactions to local anaesthetic agents and raises the threshold for convulsions. In other words, regional anaesthesia helps to avoid the complications of general anaesthesia and vice versa.In paediatric centres where regional anaesthesia is regularly practised, surgeons have begun to see it in its proper perspective and they are increasingly prepared to leave the choice of technique to the anaesthetist. This presupposes, of course, that the paediatric anaesthetist has acquired the necessary experience in adults before embarking on regional blocks in children.

For the purposes of deciding on whether to combine general and regional anaesthesia, children may be divided into two groups:

1. Pre-school age children or up to 6 or 7 years
2. Children of school age or over 7 years

Children in the first group will practically always require light general anaesthesia both for the performance of the block and for the duration of surgery. Children in the second group may tolerate the block and the surgery without the need of general anaesthesia, but this will depend on the temperament of the child and the nature of the procedure. Since general anaesthesia may be required at any stage in any child, the pre-operative assessment and preparation, which includes fasting and other precautions, is identical for both groups. The only exception here is the very much older child of equable temperament who has perhaps received, and appreciated, regional anaesthesia in the past. In such a case, unsupplemented regional block can be firmly planned and adhered to.

History

Previous personal and family history, together with a physical examination, are the cornerstones of preoperative assessment and preparation for both general and regional anaesthesia. Only when this information is available is it possible to select the best technique (general or regional anaesthesia alone or in combination), bearing in mind the needs of the child and the operation to be performed.

When regional anaesthesia is being considered, certain details are of particular importance. A history of convulsions means that great caution is required because the local anaesthetic agent may trigger an attack at comparatively low plasma concentrations. In such cases an increased dose of a preoperative sedative with an anticonvulsant action would be indicated.

A history of eczema, asthma and intolerance to cow's milk and sugars raises the possibility that the child may be allergic to drugs and adhesives. In this context it should be said that true allergy to local anaesthetics - with the exception of the ester types - is extremely rare.

Epistaxis and previous excessive blood loss, especially after dental extractions, the intake of salicylates and, possibly, anticoagulants should alert the anaesthetist to the possibility of a coagulation disorder.

Any unusual or persistent headache should be investigated to exclude raised intracranial pressure if central blocks are being considered.

A family history of neuromuscular disease may lead the anaesthetist to suspect malignant hyperpyrexia and suggest the use of a regional technique. When a child is suffering from pre-existing disease of the nervous system or when some deficit in sensory or motor function is suspected, its extent must be assessed by thorough neurological examination by a specialist in this field and his complete findings must be carefully recorded. Regional anaesthesia should only be performed in these patients if there is a clear indication, and the benefits should outweigh the possible complications. A full explanation should be given to the parents and to the child if he is old enough to understand.

During preoperative evaluation, the opportunity should be taken to note the psychological development and maturity of the child because this may influence the anaesthetist in his choice of technique. When a child belongs to the "school age or over 7 years" group and is to have unsupplemented regional anaesthesia, he must be given a clear description of what to expect, but the anaesthetist should avoid frightening words like 'needles' and "injections" (see p. 61). A separate, full explanation should also be given to the parents and agreement reached with them on whether they are to accompany their child to the anaesthetic room. The presence of parents at the induction of anaesthesia is often helpful, but each case should be decided on its merits.

When a child is in pain, he will much more readily accept a regional block when told that this will bring him relief. A "three-in-one" block for a fractured femur is a good example. If the regional technique is to be combined with general anaesthesia, the method of induction can be discussed at this visit.

The preoperative visit is the most suitable time to mention the motor block and paraesthesiae which may follow regional anaesthesia. In fact, this constitutes no significant problem if low concentrations of local anaesthetic are used, but it is always better to warn the child beforehand of this postoperative possibility so that the symptoms do not alarm and surprise him.

Physical examination

On physical examination, there are certain points of particular interest to the anaesthetist planning a regional anaesthetic. For a brachial plexus block, he should note the shape, size and mobility of the neck. If he intends to use the axillary approach, he should be sure that the arm can be abducted at the shoulder and the axillary artery palpated. If a central block is planned, the bones of the spine should be examined. Spinal deformities, such as scoliosis and kyphosis, may make epidural and spinal blocks difficult and may require special investigations as well as a different anatomical approach. Spina bifida occulta is a contraindication to the insertion of a needle in this area. This condition may be suspected if a tuft of hair, a deep dimple or a "wine stain" is visible in the lumbosacral region. Skin infection at the site of injection is an absolute contraindication to any form of regional anaesthesia.

Routine laboratory tests are performed as indicated for any child undergoing general anaesthesia and surgery. However, the coagulation profile may be of special interest to the anaesthetist planning a regional block, particularly if prematurity or the previous medical or family history suggests that this may be abnormal. Some anaesthetists feel that coagulation should always be investigated. They argue that adequate information about it is simply not available from the history in infants and young children.

Premedication

Satisfactory sedation prior to regional block in children is of prime importance. The oral preparation of diazepam, given in a dose of $0.2mg.kg^{-1}$ up to a maximum of 10mg is one of the most useful agents and should be given at least one hour before the block. Children premedicated with this regime are surprisingly calm, yet they are also conversational and able to cooperate with the anaesthetist and monitor paraesthesiae. The relatively large dose of diazepam has the advantage that it raises the threshold for convulsions, though this should not be used as licence for overdosage with local anaesthetic and poor technique. Light general anaesthesia may be more suitable than sedation in some cases. When the anaesthetist is deciding between sedation or anaesthesia, his most important consideration must be that the performance of a regional block by force and restraint is unacceptable. Not only is it distressing and psychologically damaging to the child, but it also makes the block more difficult and dangerous to perform.

Preparation for the block

The equipment required for regional blocks is dealt with on p. 68. It must of course be sterile. The skin must be disinfected and draped, and the anaesthetist should wear sterile gloves for most blocks. Some procedures even require full gowning. The conduct of the staff has been described in detail on page 61. Once the patient arrives in the anaesthetic or operating room, the anaesthetist should renew friendly, reassuring and calming contact with him. The child should feel that he is entering into a happy, relaxed, quiet atmosphere in which anaesthesia is part of the routine and not a "big deal". Where light general anaesthesia is planned prior to the block, it should be started straight away so the child is not kept waiting. Where paraesthesiae are to be elicited the anaesthetist should remind the patient about what he will feel and what is required of him.

During the search for paraesthesiae, he should be in constant verbal contact with the child, and an assistant holding the child's hand during a brachial plexus block may well feel a sudden contraction when nerve contact is made. At other times however, incessant questioning about paraesthesiae and subjective sensations is only confusing. The anaesthetist must tell the child what to expect before each stage in the procedure but he must choose his words carefully. "Cool" is a suitable word to use before application of the skin preparation and "a little scratch" is a good euphemism for an injection. Throughout the procedure the anaesthetist should constantly encourage the child and let him know how much he is helping everybody with his cooperation.

Testing for the effect of the block should not be done before analgesia can reasonably be expected. Constant testing is very disturbing. If a needle is used, care should be taken that it does not leave marks as these may be distressing to the child, the parents and even the surgeon. Firm pinching gives good information about surgical analgesia and does not leave marks.

Monitoring

Clinical observation of the patient is the most valuable method of monitoring a regional block and there is really no mechanical substitute for this. Changes in skin colour, such as cyanosis and pallor, and in respiratory rate and depth are important. Sudden talkativeness and confusion in the awake child may indicate systemic local anaesthetic toxicity. The size and shape of the pupils require special attention from the time the block has been performed until it is fully established.

Other mandatory monitoring aids are the same as for general anaesthesia and include a precordial stethoscope, sphygmomanometer and electrocardiogram with acoustic rate monitor. For longer operations, an oesophageal or rectal temperature probe is recommended for measuring core temperature.

Intravenous infusion

An intravenous line must be established as soon as the patient is asleep. In the very exceptional case in whom the veins are extremely poor, it is justifiable to perform the block first and insert a cannula once vasodilatation has occurred in the affected part. The equipment should be out of sight when the child enters the anaesthetic room.

General Anaesthesia

The combination of light general anaesthesia with regional anaesthesia is almost ideal in paediatric practice. It allows the block to be performed under good conditions, it renders the patient oblivious to the disturbing surroundings of the operating room, and it enables the anaesthetist to ventilate the patient artificially if this is clinically required. Yet, almost all the advantages of regional anaesthesia are retained. Of course, all the procedures, investigations, premedication and monitoring ordinarily required for general anaesthesia have to be carried out, as pointed out earlier, and a competent assistant is required to supervise the general anaesthetic while the anaesthetist is performing the block.

General anaesthesia may be induced by any of the usual methods. Nitrous oxide, oxygen and halothane, enflurane or isoflurane can be given by mask. 0.5% halothane or 1% enflurane in a mixture of 50% nitrous oxide and oxygen is sufficient to maintain a light level of anaesthesia, allowing tolerance of an endotracheal tube and mechanical ventilation. IV or IM induction with ketamine is also possible.

The nature and duration of the surgery, the intra-operative position of the patient and the adverse effect of these factors on pulmonary function, especially in the very young, usually require that the trachea is intubated. Intubation decreases the dead space volume by approximately half, although the intrapulmonary dead space appears very similar in awake and anaesthetized spontaneously-breathing children. For long operations, mechanical ventilation is preferred because it reduces the amount of energy expended on the work of breathing. Humidification of inspired gases is desirable during controlled ventilation because it not only prevents the drying of pulmonary secretions, but also assists in the maintenance of core temperature and in the preservation of normal plasma pH - acidosis increases the toxicity of local anaesthetics.

If an intravenous line has already been established, it can be used for the administration of thiopentone or one of the other suitable induction agents. Ketamine is a very convenient drug because it allows the establishment of an intravenous line as well as the positioning for, and performance of, the block. It can be given intramuscularly in a dose of 4- 5mg.kg^{-1} or rectally in a dose of 10 - 12mg.kg^{-1}.

Intubation may be indicated for clinical reasons such as a full stomach, an upper abdominal procedure, a bizarre operating position, a prolonged operation or elective artificial ventilation. In such cases, it may be performed immediately after induction under topical local anaesthetic spray or with the aid of a short-acting muscle relaxant.

Once the airway has been secured, with a mask or tube, the patient is ready for the block and is positioned accordingly. This is a critical moment for the airway, even in the intubated child, and special attention has to be paid to it. The same applies after the block when the child is returned to the supine or placed in the operating position. Restraints are firmly applied above the knees, and both arms have to be well secured so that involuntary movements under light general anaesthesia do not disturb the surgeon or contaminate the operative field. This is also the time to apply padding where necessary to protect superficially-running nerves which may be damaged by pressure, and to check for harmful

positions such as hyperextension.

While waiting for the block to become effective, the surgical team is allowed to disinfect the skin and even to start surgery. During this period, the patient is kept anaesthetised in the usual way with normal concentrations of halothane or enflurane or small increments of ketamine. When sufficient time has elapsed for the block to be effective, the concentration of halothane or enflurane is reduced and the increments of ketamine are withheld. A rise in pulse rate and blood pressure, and other signs of pain, such as increase in respiratory rate, dilatation of the pupils and defensive move-ments, indicate that the block is still incomplete or has failed. In the latter case, general anaesthesia is continued in the normal fashion and becomes fully effective within a few minutes. If none of the above symptoms occur, analgesia from the block may be assumed complete, and general anaesthesia is continued at a reduced concentration, resulting in "balanced anaesthesia"in which the inhalation agent produces amnesia, permits toleration of the endotracheal tube and prevents movement of the patient, and the block supplies the analgesia and muscle relaxation. In some cases, the inhalation agent can be discontinued altogether. Visceral impulses, which occasionally come through despite an effective block, may be obtunded by small doses of ketamine. With such a light general anaesthetic, it must be remembered that any inadvertent stimulation in unblocked parts of the body will cause defensive reactions by the child.

Artifical ventilation is applied purely on clinical grounds. If coughing occurs or transient relaxation is required, a small dose of a short-acting muscle relaxant is given and the child is artificially ventilated until the agent has worn off. Non- depolarising muscle relaxants , which sometimes result in the need for postoperative ventilation, are not usually necessary.

Unsupplemented regional anaesthesia

As already mentioned, this approach can only be undertaken in the older child, but special attention has still to be paid to the psychological problems which may occur when a conscious child comes into contact with the frightening noises and equipment in the operating room. The anaesthetist, who is by now the child's familiar "friend", can provide constant reassurance by his uninterrupted presence, and he can help to distract the child during the operation by telling stories, playing word games and questioning him about his interests and hobbies. The verbal contact should be kept up all the time, but additional sedation may still be needed inspite of this. Small increments of an intravenous benzo-diazepine are very useful and may promote sleep. Only when the child is asleep may the anaes-thetist cease the verbal contact.

Any regional block may fail for many reasons, and this possibility has to be taken into account. If a block fails, it is important, both for the patient's comfort and for the anaesthetist's relationship with the surgeon, to be able to proceed to a general anaesthetic technique at a moment's notice. Appropriate drugs must therefore be drawn up preoperatively. Intravenous ketamine will establish adequate analgesia in slightly less than one minute and it lasts at least 10 minutes. Surgery will therefore only be delayed for a matter of seconds and the operating room schedule will not be disrupted. With a partially effective block, $0.3 - 0.4$mg.kg^{-1} of ketamine may suffice. In a case of complete failure, 1mg.kg^{-1}, followed by immediate induction of inhalation anaesthesia, will be necessary.

Post-operative follow-up
After operation, the anaesthetist is responsible for visiting the child to assess the quality of post-operative analgesia, to make adjustments where necessary and to ensure that no complications have occured.

Possible complications
Damage to tissues
This may take several forms. Nerves and muscles may be damaged due either to faulty positioning or to surgical trauma. Since the former is an anaesthetic responsibility and the latter a surgical one, such damage can be the cause of dispute between the two teams. Intraneural injection of the local anaesthetic will cause direct damage to the nerve fibres, but a nerve may also be damaged extraneurally if the injection pressure around it remains high or if the drug itself is irritant. The child must be protected, during and after operation, from excessive heat from electric blankets and hot water bottles, and burns may occur over

anaesthetised areas. Similarly, the effects of pressure may go unnoticed and ulceration may develop over bony points.

Headache
Headache may follow spinal and, occasionally, epidural anaesthesia. In such cases, it is important to eliminate septic and aseptic meningitis as a cause.

Paraplegia and cauda equina syndrome
This is the major neurological complication of spinal and epidural anaesthesia, but it is fortunately extremely rare and no case has yet been described in a child.

The tight plaster cast
It should be remembered that the usual symptom of pain may be masked by residual analgesia when regional anaesthesia has been used, and it is important to look out for this and other simple but potentially dangerous complications.

Suggested reading
1. Brown TCK, Fisk GC (1979) Anaesthesia for Children. Blackwell Scientific Publications
2. Gregory GA (1983) Pediatric Anesthesia. Churchill Livingstone
3. Hatch DJ, Sumner E (1985) Paediatric Anaesthesia. Clinics in Anesthesiology. WB Saunders Vol. 3 No. 3
4. Steward DJ (1979) Manual of Pediatric Anesthesia. Churchill Livingstone

Equipment

Marie Madeleine Delleur

Introduction

When the anaesthetist is choosing the equipment and materials for use during the management of anaesthesia, his first consideration must be the safety and well-being of the child.

Where regional anaesthesia is concerned, the equipment is not limited simply to that required for performance of the block. It must also include the means for inducing and maintaining general anaesthesia and for treating extensive sympathetic block, local anaesthetic toxicity and any other complications which may occur. When regional anaesthesia was first practised in children, no suitable equipment was available and the anaesthetist had to improvise. However, equipment specially designed for paediatric use is now available so blocks can be performed more easily and with less risk of complications

General anaesthesia

The safety of the child depends ultimately on the vigilance of the anaesthetist. All equipment, including monitoring for general anaesthesia, must be appropriate for the age and condition of the child because general anaesthesia may be necessary to supplement an inadequate block or replace a failed one.

Intravenous equipment

Intravenous access should be secured before a regional block is performed in a child. Small catheters are usually used, ranging in size from 18 to 25G. Butterfly needles are less satisfactory because they are liable to cut out of the vein at the slightest movement. All needles and catheters must be securely fixed.

Intravenous electrolyte and glucose solutions are identical with those normally used during paediatric anaesthesia.

Temperature maintenance

The maintenance of normal body temperature is especially important in children and its supervision should be carried out as usual.

Emergency drugs

When an emergency arises and the anaesthetist is working under stress, mistakes can easily occur so it is recommended that a chart, giving drug dosages in millilitres of solution per kilogram body weight, is readily available.

Mean recommended doses intravenously are:

atropine:	$0.02mg.kg^{-1}$
	min 0.1mg
adrenaline:	$10\mu g.kg^{-1}$
	($0.1ml.kg^{-1}$ of 1 in
	10.000 solution
sodium bicarbonate:	$1mmol.kg^{-1}$
	$1ml.kg^{-1}$ of
	8.4% solution
calcium chloride:	$5-10mg.kg^{-1}$
	$0.3ml.kg^{-1}$ of
	10% solution
calcium gluconate:	$30mg.kg^{-1}$
	$1ml.kg^{-1}$ of
	10% solution
isoprenaline infusion:	0.05 to
	$0.1\mu g.kg^{-1}.min^{-1}$
dopamine infusion:	$1-5\mu g.kg^{-1}.min^{-1}$
frusemide:	$1mg.kg^{-1}$
diazepam:	$0.1-0.2mg.kg^{-1}$
hydrocortisone:	$0.1mg.kg^{-1}$
dexamethasone:	$0.2mg.kg^{-1}$

Regional anaesthesia

This section outlines the equipment most commonly used for paediatric regional anaesthesia. It is best to have this equipment ready assembled and stored on a trolley kept specially for the purpose. This saves time and ensures that everything is at hand. The following materials should be available:

sterile gloves of different sizes
sterile towels and drapes
skin cleaning solutions (which should be
    compatible with the solutions to be used
    by the surgeon)
adhesive tape and dressings
needles and catheters, either individually packed
    or incorporated in disposable kits
1ml, 5ml, 10ml and 20ml syringes for local
    anaesthetic injection. These syringes
    should be distinguished by a coloured
    marker to avoid any confusion with those
    used for general anaesthesia.
micropore filters with a pore size of 0.22μm,
    capable of trapping bacteria and small
    particles such as glass, etc.
local anaesthetic solutions with and without
    adrenaline.
drugs for emergency use (see earlier in this
    chapter)
standard sterile instrument tray to include:

> 1 bowl for skin cleaning solution
> swabs and swab-holding forceps
> 1 towel
> 1 glass container for the anaesthetic
>   solution
> 20ml vial of normal saline solution
> 2 x 21G needles
> 1 x 18G needle for perforation of the skin
> 3ml, 5ml and 10ml glass syringes or
>   special plastic syringes (Portex) for
>   identification of the epidural space
> micropore filter straw (Burron Medical -
>   FS 5000) for drawing up the local
>   anaesthetic
> a pair of scissors
> an ampoule file.

Packing and sterilisation

The anaesthetist must be able to rely on the sterility of the materials he uses. Disposable products, for use once only, are obviously ideal because sterility is guaranteed by the manufacturer. Sterilisation is usually carried out by exposure to ethylene oxide or gamma radiation. The expiry date is printed on each pack and this must be checked before use.

Alternatively, epidural packs can be prepared in the hospital's sterile department. Costs can be reduced if needles and syringes can be used several times, but strict attention must be given to sterility, and catheters <u>must</u> <u>not</u> <u>be</u> <u>re-used</u>. Needles and syringes should be cleansed by scrubbing with water, but soap and detergent should never be used as these agents may cause neural damage (5). The equipment should be thoroughly rinsed and well dried before being packed.

Tuohy needles should be separated from their stylets for the sterilisation process. A mark made on each needle and its stylet will ensure that they can be correctly re-united after sterilisation. This is important because it is dangerous to use a Tuohy needle with a stylet which does not extend to the needle tip.

Wrapped epidural trays are sterilised in a steam autoclave and sterilisation indicators should be placed inside and outside the pack which should be marked with the date of sterilisation and the name of the person responsible for the procedure.

Local anaesthetic solutions should not be included in block trays because their potency may be reduced by autoclave heat. For central blocks, local anaesthetic in multiple-dose bottles should not be used owing to the risk of contamination from repeated use. The use of preservative-free solutions in snap ampoules and of micropore filter straws is recommended.

Single-shot caudal block

Children under 1 year

Three different needles are suitable: 23 and 25G short bevel Butterfly needles may be used. However, there is a danger that an infant's soft bone may be penetrated more easily with these small sizes than with the ordinary 20G needle or with one specially designed for paediatric lumbar puncture.

Children over 1 year

The choice lies between the 20G short bevel paediatric lumbar puncture needle, the 18 or 20G intravenous cannulae, or Hody's 18G, thin-walled needle (photo 2). Some anaesthetists prefer the larger 18 or 20G needles because they give a better "feel" on puncturing the sacrococcygeal ligament (6).

Continuous caudal block

The anaesthetist must check, before performing the block, that the catheter will pass down the needle. Hody's needle and the 18 or 20G plastic or teflon intravenous cannula (photo 2) are suitable. Catheters are made in 18, 19, 20 and 24G sizes, and are available with and without stylet (see epidural chapter).

Epidural block

The "ideal" epidural needle should have the following features (7):

a well-fitting stylet
a short, directional bevel with rounded edges
a terminal orifice.

It should be available in a variety of gauges so that the anaesthetist can select the smallest size appropriate for the case. These features contribute towards safe epidural puncture and help to avoid the following undesirable complications:

1. Implantation of skin fragments into the epidural space. This can occur if the stylet does not completely occlude the needle orifice.

2. Puncture of the dura and blood vessels. The contoured bevel of the Tuohy needle is designed to minimise this and it also ensures that the catheter emerges at an angle, thus helping its passage into the epidural space. However, a catheter, once inserted, must never be withdrawn through the needle because it can be sheared off or transected by the bevel. If it is necessary to withdraw the catheter, the needle must also be withdrawn at the same rate.

The paediatric Tuohy needle differs from the adult version in a number of ways. It is shorter - a length of 5cm is suitable for children and it prevents increased lever action when it approaches the epidural space. It is graduated in

0.5cm rather than 1cm intervals. This is more appropriate when the distance between the skin and the space is small. Different gauges are now available.

Choice of needle for single-shot technique

Up to the age of 2 years

The following needles are suitable:
short bevel 23G Butterfly
20G Tuohy needle (see above)

Between 2 and 8 years

20, 19 or 18G Tuohy needles may be used. For the beginner, the largest (18) gauge gives the best "feel" of the ligament, but of course a large hole is made if the dura is accidentally punctured.

Over 8 years old

The standard needle is the 18G Tuohy. The 17G may be more suitable in the older or obese child, and the 18G in the adolescent where the lateral approach may have to be used.

Choice of catheter for continuous technique

The "ideal" catheter represents a compromise between conflicting requirements (7).

Rigidity

The catheter should be rigid enough to pass through the Tuohy needle, but not so rigid that it causes damage in the epidural space. The insertion of a stylet increases rigidity of the very small (24G) catheters and this is helpful for passing the catheter through the needle. However, certain conditions must be fulfilled when a stylet is used. It must be shorter than the catheter so that there is no risk of it protruding beyond the catheter tip. It must always be withdrawn before the catheter enters the epidural space - its role is solely to facilitate the passage of the catheter down the needle. For this reason, a stylet is only safe when used with a Tuohy needle, since the contoured bevel makes it obvious when the catheter has reached the tip.

Strength and resistance

The catheter should be strong enough to withstand moderate tensile force (8) so that it does not break on removal. On the other hand, the lumen must be as large as possible to reduce the resistance to injection or infusion.

Tissue reaction

The catheter should be manufactured from biologically inert material so that it can, if necessary, be left in the epidural space for long periods without causing tissue reaction. Poly-urethane is very good from this point of view (9).

Other features

The tip is the part of the catheter most likely to cause damage, and its design is important. It should be smooth and rounded. The use of catheters with a blind end and multiple lateral holes is to be discouraged for a number of reasons. On aspiration the lateral openings tend to get occluded by tissue, in particular the walls of vessels, thus impeding the recognition of an intravascular position of the catheter. The distal holes may be in the subarachnoid space while the proximal ones are in the epidural space. Perforation of the dura may therefore not be recognised and on injection a total spinal may result. Furthermore, cases have been described where the catheter on removal has broken at the site of the lateral holes. Therefore it appears wise to use simple catheters with a single terminal hole.

The catheter should be graduated. This enables the anaesthetist to know the length which has been inserted. Catheters with radio-opaque lining are not necessary and make recognition of returning blood difficult. If verification of the catheter's position is required, radio-opaque solution can be injected.

Catheter size, needle gauge and age of patient

Information about the specification of catheters varies with different manufacturers. In some cases, both internal and external diameters are given, whereas in others, only the external diameter is quoted, with the gauge of the Tuohy needle through which it will pass (Table 8.). In practice, it is best to choose the largest external diameter compatible with the needle to be used. Internal diameters sometimes vary between catheters of the same external diameter and in such cases the catheter with the largest internal diameter should be chosen in order that the pressure required for injection or infusion is minimal. In every case, the anaesthetist must check, before he starts the block, that the catheter fits the needle and is patent.

For children from 1 to 4 years, in whom a 20 or 19G Tuohy needle is used, catheters with an external diameter between 0.5 and 0.8mm are required. For those over 4 years, in whom a 19 or 18G Tuohy needle is used, external diameters between 0.7 and 1mm are suitable. In special cases, such as the older or obese child, a 17G Tuohy needle may be needed and a catheter with an external diameter of 1 to 1.1mm can then be used.

Fixation

The practice of spraying the entry site of the catheter with an aerosol solution such as Nobecutane is to be discouraged because the plastic of the catheter can be denatured and even dissolved by these solutions.

Øext o Øint/Øext	Gauge	Length mm	Extremity	Mandrin	Ext Grad.	Xray Opacity	Material	Trade-Mark	Ref.
1,05	16 G	1000	3 lateral holes	No	X	Yes and No	Polyamide without Plastifiant	Braun-Melsungen Perifix	415325/8 451310/0
1,1	16 G	900	3 lateral holes	No No	X X	No No	Clear Nylon	Portex	100/382/116
0,5/1	19 G	900	No lateral hole	Yes	X	Yes	Polyethylene	Vygon	185/10
0,5/1	19 G	900	No lateral hole	No	X	Yes	Polyethylene	Vygon	186/10
0,5/1	19 G	900	3 lateral holes	No	X	No	Nylon	Vermeed	59/730
0,63/1	18 G	918	No lateral hole	No	X	Yes	Rilsan	Abbott	E622
0,9	18 G	900	3 lateral holes	No	X	No	Clear Nylon	Portex	100/394/118
0,85	18 G	1000	3 lateral holes	No	X	Yes and No	Polyamide without Plastifiant	Braun-Melsungen Perifix	415315/0
0,5/0,8	20 G	900	3 lateral holes	No	X	No	Nylon	Vermed	59/731
0,5/0,7	19 G	450	No lateral holes	Yes	X	Yes	Polyurethane	Vermed	60810
0,63	19 G	900	No lateral hole	No	X	No	Clear Nylon	Portex	139/382 219/075
0,3/0,6	-	400	No lateral hole	Yes	X	Yes	Polyurethane	Vygon	8128506
0,2/0,5	24 G	300 and 350	No lateral hole	Yes	X	Yes	Polyurethane	Vermed	63815

Table 8.

Spinal block

Several needles are suitable, depending on the age of the child. For children under 2 years, the short bevel 25G Butterfly may be used. For older patients, a range of paediatric lumbar puncture needles, with stylet, is available (see Table 9.). The needle should be rigid enough not to bend during insertion. Some needles, such as the "pencil"-tipped Whiteacre, are designed to separate the fibres of the dura instead of cutting them. This minimises the outflow of cerebro-spinal fluid and reduces the risk of headache (10). A similar effect can be obtained with needles of conventional design if the tip is introduced with its bevel parallel to the longitudinally-running dural fibres.

Ext. mm	Diam. Gauge	Length mm	Manufacturer	Ref.
	26		Braun Melsungen	
45/100	26	90	Becton Dickinson	5164
5/10	25	40	Vygon	SVP
	64		Sherwood (Diamant tip)	
	90		Becton Dickinson	5180
7/10	22	40	Sherwood	
	40		Becton Dickinson	5161
	64		Becton Dickinson	5074

Stylet of the percutaneous catheters 24 or 25G = 27G needle (41/100)

Table 9. Spinal anaesthesia needles

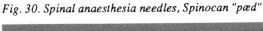

Fig. 30. Spinal anaesthesia needles, Spinocan "pæd"

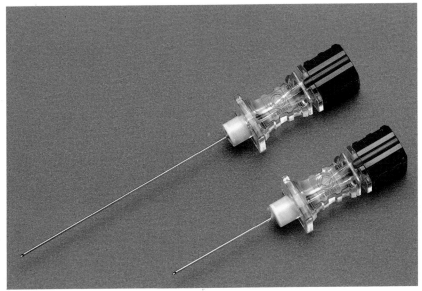

73

Peripheral nerve blocks

Short-bevel needles are a prerequisite for these blocks. They are available as individual items and as short-bevel Butterfly needles. Standard extension tubing may be connected to them. The choice of needle gauge will depend on the block and the size of the child. For example, penile block can be performed with a 25G. For axillary and subclavicular blocks, the size will depend on the age of the child:

Up to 2 years:	24 or 23G
2 to 4 years:	20G
Over 4 years:	19 or 20G.

Since most of these blocks are performed on anaesthetised children, paraesthesias cannot be obtained and a nerve stimulator is therefore necessary. The best stimulators deliver a short pulse (40 microseconds) combined with a low maximum current limited to 3mA. Under these conditions, the nerve can only be stimulated when the tip of the sheathed needle connected to the stimulator is very close to the nerve. At a distance of 1cm from the nerve, there will be no response at all (11).

More recently, B. Braun-Melsungen, in Germany, has manufactured a nerve stimulator which produces currents from 0.2 to 0.5mA in increments of 0.1mA. It also delivers a pulse of very short duration - 0.1msec instead of the more usual 1msec. As a result, motor fibres can be selectively stimulated without unpleasant sensory effects being caused. As with the Anaestim, stimulation is only possible when the tip of the sheathed needle is within 1cm of the nerve. Nerve stimulators with a greater electrical radius require considerable manipulation of the needle for optimal paraesthesiae to be obtained.

Short bevel needles are available with a double connection (photo ?4). The teflon needle, electrically connected to the nerve stimulator, has a length of extension tubing which allows the local anaesthetic solution to be injected without moving the needle. The needle should be insulated throughout almost all its length so that the electric current is concentrated at the tip.

Summary

Regional anaesthetic techniques can be successfully and widely applied in paediatrics, but the equipment used should be specially designed for use in children. The anaesthetist should be able to select from the extensive range available, the equipment which suits him best and with which he feels most familiar.

Fig. 31.

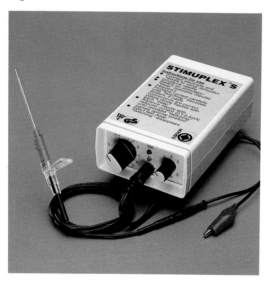

Fig. 32.

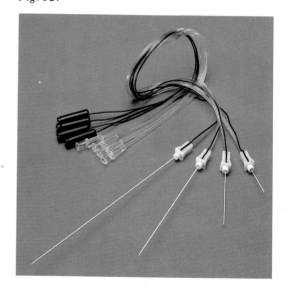

References

1. Brown TCK, Fisk GC (1979) Anaesthesia for children. Blackwell Scientific Publications

2. Gregory GA (1983) Pediatric anesthesia. Churchill Livingstone

3. Sumner E, Hatch D (1985) Clinics in Anaesthesiology. Saunders Company. Vol 3 No 3

4. Steward DJ (1985) Manual of pediatric anesthesia. Churchill Livingstone

5. Winkelman, NW (1952) Neurologic symptoms following accidental intraspinal detergent injection. Neurology 2:284

6. Schulte Steinberg O (1988) Neural blockade for pediatric surgery. In Neural Blockade, edited by Cousins MJ, Bridenbaugh PO, Philadelphia JB. Lippincott 676

7. Bromage PR (1978) Epidural analgesia. Philadelphia, Saunders

8. Belatti RG, Fromme GA, Danielson DR (1985) Relative resistance to shearing of commercially available epidural catheters versus available epidural needles in Equipment, Monitoring and Engineering - Neurosciences - Posters Anesthesiology

9. Curelaru I, Gustavsson B, Hultman E, Jondmundsson E, Linder LE, Stefansson T and Stenquist O (1984) Material thrombogenicity in central venous catheterization III. A comparison between soft polyvinylchloride and soft polyurethane elastomer, long, antebrachial catheters. Acta Anaesth Scand 28:204

10. Drazen N, Mihic (1985) Postspinal headache and relationship of needle bevel to longitudinal dural fibers. Regional anesthesia, Vol 10, no 2:76

11. Gribromont B. (in publication). Features of nerve stimulators as used in loco-regional anaesthesia

II. Techniques

Introduction to epidural anaesthesia

Ottheinz Schulte Steinberg

For decades, caudal anaesthesia has been the only form of epidural practised in children although, as has been pointed out in the History chapter page 13, epidural anaesthesia can be used at several levels. As the advantages of combining general anaesthesia with regional blocks became more widely appreciated, these other approaches to the epidural space have become popular as well. It is now recognised that epidural anaesthesia has a definite place in paediatrics. The indications are similar to those in adults and the benefits have been discussed in General Principles and Benefits page 9.

..The absolute contraindications, which are the same for all central blocks, are local infection of the skin at the site of needle puncture, coagulopathies and uncorrected hypovolaemia. Degenerative neuropathies and spinal diseases have also been regarded as contraindications, but modern opinion does not always agree with this.

Epidural anaesthesia in children should only be attempted by anaesthetists who have extensive experience with these techniques in adults. The incidence of complications is inversely proportional to the experience of the anaesthetist. The equipment used should be specially designed for children. An intravenous line must first be established. In almost every case the block will need to be performed under light general anaesthesia with inhalational agents, or intra-venous or intramuscular ketamine. This applies for epidural blocks below the end of the spinal cord.

Blocks above L4 in the newborn and above L2 after the first year and in particular thoracic epidural blocks require a patient who will react when the needle approaches the cord. Therefore general anaesthesia should be limited exclusively to very unusual circumstances, when there is no other solution to a special problem.

Expertise in paediatric epidural anaesthesia is of prime importance. Written informed consent of the parents should be obtained and inserted into the record of the child. The surgeon should be notified. A written note in the record outlining the "real benefit" of the technique is important in case of medio-legal implications.

Usually lumbar epidural anaesthesia will suffice. In smaller infants a thoracic epidural block can mostly be established by the caudal approach. Because of the greater stability provided, the block is almost always performed in the lateral position. While the block is being performed, a reliable assistant must pay special attention not only to the general anaesthetic, but especially to the airway. This applies particularly when the child's position is changed even if he has been intubated.

Disinfection of the skin, as described previously, is performed after the child has been positioned, and the epidural equipment is prepared afterwards so that the skin has time to dry. The risk of introducing liquid disinfectant when the needle is inserted is thereby eliminated.

Since aspiration tests are unreliable, a test dose with an adrenaline-containing local anaesthetic solution should be given in all epidural techniques. During the minute after injection, the ECG is observed for tachycardia and/or arrhythmias. These indicate that the catheter tip lies intravascularly. Also, the blood pressure is measured at this time for any significant alterations. Finally, when a continuous technique is being used, the catheter is held below the level of the patient after injection of the test dose, and observed for any flowback of blood or cerebrospinal fluid under gravity.

Drugs

The drugs used for all types of epidural anaesthesia are the same. Lidocaine and mepivacaine (both 1%) for short procedures and bupivacaine 0.25% for longer ones are used for infants and small children. When used in combination with general anaesthesia, bupivacaine will last 60-90 minutes. If adrenaline is added, the duration can be extended to 90-120 minutes. For intra-abdominal procedures, relaxation can be obtained by increasing the concentration of lidocaine or mepivacaine to 1.5% and bupivacaine to 0.375% in this age group. For older children, 2% lidocaine, 2% mepivacaine and 0.5% bupivacaine are needed, particularly if relaxation is wanted.

The use of 0.75% bupivacaine for profound relaxation and motor block is not recommended in children because of the danger that toxic concentrations may be reached rapidly. If such relaxation is required, etidocaine 0.75%-1% may be added to the solution, but this mixture is unsuitable for single-shot caudal block, and for other techniques it should be limited to the earlier stages of surgery because of the long duration of action of etidocaine. If etidocaine is not available, 2% lidocaine with adrenaline is an alternative. The adrenaline increases the relaxant effect considerably.

The addition of adrenaline, 1 in 200.000, to local anaesthetic solutions increases their duration of action, especially in very young children. A recent study by Murat et al, in which she used 0.25% bupivacaine, showed that with adrenaline the time between top-ups was increased by 47% in children under 2 years, by 25% in those between 2 and 8 years, and by 12% in those over 8 years (1)(Fig. 33.). These results are similar to those reported by Warner who used bupivacaine by the caudal route for postoperative pain relief

and suggested that the effect was due to a decrease in the vascular uptake of the local anaesthetic and perhaps also to the more profound block produced by adrenaline in young children (2). The relative lack of epidural fat in children may well be responsible for the increased effect of adrenaline with the highly lipid soluble bupivacaine.

This prolongation of action is an important reason for recommending adrenaline 1 in 200.000 because it reduces the number and frequency of top-up injections and, hence, the total dose of local anaesthetic required during and after surgery. Adrenaline can induce tachycardia so it is best avoided in cardiac patients in whom this may be undesirable, but there are no other contraindications.

Small volumes of local anaesthetic will be adequate if the level of epidural puncture is carefully matched to the area involved in the surgery. The use of an epidural catheter allows a minimal volume to be injected initially. If this dose proves insufficient at the time of skin incision, supplementary doses can easily be given until adequate analgesia has been obtained.

There are two approaches to the timing of top-up injections. They may be given regularly, the intervals being determined by the pharmacolo-

Fig. 33. Shows the prolongation of analgesia by the addition of adrenaline to bupivacaine versus plain bupivacaine in epidural application (1). I Murat et al (1987) Br J Anaesth

Fig. 34. Pharmacokinetics of bupivacaine 0.25% with adrenaline, in 5 children aged 1 to 7 (5). I Murat et al (1988) Eur J Anaesth

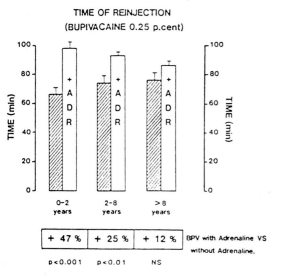

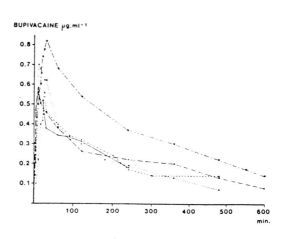

79

gical properties and the known duration of action of the drug; or they may be given in response to changes in heart rate, pupillary dilatation or systolic blood pressure, which occur in the absence of any obvious surgical cause such as uncorrected blood loss. The presence or absence of adrenaline, the concentration of local anaesthetic used and the age of the child all influence the time interval between top-ups. The mean interval for bupivacaine with adrenaline 1 in 200.000 in children is about 110 minutes and about 70 minutes for the plain solution (1-5).

The top-up interval decreases as age increases because pharmacokinetic factors vary with age (4). As with adults, the recommended top-up dose is half the initial dose. During the postoperative period 0.125%-0.25% bupivacaine is sufficient to provide pain control. If recommended doses are adhered to, peak plasma concentrations are low and the safety margin is very wide compared with adults, in whom concentrations of 4µg/ml may be regarded as toxic. When 0.25% bupivacaine (Fig. 34.) with adrenaline 1 in 200.000 is injected epidurally in a dose of 0.75ml/kg, the peak plasma concentration is only 0.64 µg/ml (+ or - 0.05)(5).

Absorption half life is short (6). The apparent volume of distribution decreases as age increases. In children between 1 and 6 years it is three times greater than in adults (7).

References

1. Murat I, Delleur MM, Esteve C, Egu JF Raynaud P, Saint-Maurice C (1987) Continuous epidural anaesthesia in children: clinical and haemodynamic implications. Br J Anaesth 59:1441

2. Warner MA, Kunkel SE, Offord KO, Atchinson SR, Dawson B (1987) The effects of age, epinephrine, and operative site on duration of caudal analgesia in pediatric patients. Anesth Analg 66:995

3. Delleur MM, Murat I, Estève C, Raynaud P, Gaudiche D, Saint-Maurice C (1985) Anesthesie peridurale continue chez l'enfant de moins de deux ans. Ann Fr Anesth Reanim 4:413

4. Eyres RL, Kidd J, Oppenheim R, Brown TCK (1978) Local anaesthetic plasma levels in children. Anaesth Intens Care 6:243

5. Murat I, Montay G, Delleur MM, Estève C, Saint-Maurice C (1988) Bupivacaine pharmacokinetics during epidural anaesthesia in children. Eur J Anaesth 5:113

6. Ecoffey C, Desparmet J, Mavry M, Berdeaux A, Guidicelli JF, Saint-Maurice C (1985) Bupivacaine in Children: Pharmacokinetics following Caudal Anesthesia. Anesthesiology 63:447.

7. Mather LE, Tucker GT (1978) Pharmacokinetics and Biotransformation of Local Anesthetics. Int Anesth Clin 16:23.

Single shot caudal block

Elisabeth Giaufre

Introduction

The easiest and safest approach to the infant's epidural space is by the caudal route. If the single shot technique is correctly performed and the anatomy is normal, there is no danger of the needle penetrating the dural sac or damaging the spinal cord. This is true even for the newborn in whom these structures extend more caudad than in the adult.

Indications

The technique is suitable for surgical procedures below T10 lasting less than 90 minutes, such as inguinal hernia, perineal surgery and operations on the lower extremities. It is also suitable for orchidopexy, provided that the testes are not intra-abdominal when a higher sensory innervation is involved. It is particularly indicated for hypospadias, skin grafting and anal surgery. Bleeding, which can be profuse in these operations, can be reduced by this anaesthetic technique (1,2,3). Incarcerated inguinal hernias can often be reduced easily under caudal block and operated upon electively at a later date when normal bowel action has resumed.

Contraindications

Although there are no special contraindications, the single shot technique is unsuitable for procedures involving dermatomes above T10 because of the large quantities of local anaesthetic required (4), and operations lasting longer than about 90 minutes are likely to out-last the duration of the block. Both these situations are better managed with a caudal catheter, as described in the next chapter. Children weighing more than 30kg may be technically difficult because their anatomy and landmarks approximate to the adult, but this is not a contraindication.

Choice of drug

For single shot caudal block, the initial dose must be large enough to provide the required level of analgesia in every case, because if surgery has commenced, no additional dose can be given. On the other hand, the dose must always be well below the toxic range.

Dosage

This will depend upon the level of sensory block required, but dose requirements generally depend on several other factors. Bromage (5) has emphasised the importance of the concept of the mass of drug required to anaesthetize one segment, and Usubiaga (6) has studied pressure changes which take place in the epidural space at and immediately after the time of injection and which may influence the spread of local anaesthetic within the space. Schulte Steinberg (7) has shown that the volume of drug needed to anaesthetize one segment correlates best with age, but also very closely with weight and height. The dose of 0.1ml per segment per year of age suggested by

Fig. 35. Regression line obtained from studies with 1% Lidocaine, 1% Mepivacaine 0.25% Bupivacaine and 95% confidence lines. n=152

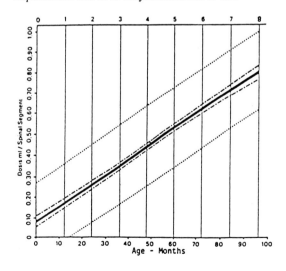

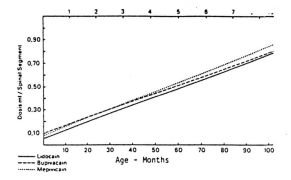

Fig. 36. *Combined regression lines of Lidocaine,*
Bupivacaine and Mepivacaine.

Schulte Steinberg (Figs 35 and 36) was based on assessment of analgesia by pin prick - a stimulus which is transmitted by C fibres, but which does not test the A delta fibres. Busoni tested both groups of fibres by severe pinching and found that considerably lower levels of analgesia were obtained. The difference in spread between the two modalities averages 4 to 6 dermatomes and the threshold of block between them appears to be considerably more extensive in children than in adults. Busoni devised a mathematical model, based on these findings (8), which gave doses higher than those recommended by Schulte

Fig. 37. *Dose requirement related to age and*
weight, from Busoni

Steinberg. For clinical purposes, in which full surgical analgesia is required, the dose should be calculated according to Busoni's diagrams (Fig 37) using 1% mepivacaine or any equipotent drug. These diagrams show that both age and weight are good predictors of the level of analgesia, and when these parameters are used for calculating dosage, there is no statistical difference between them. In neonates and infants in whom the 'age' may have been obstetrically determined, weight is the best guide, whereas age is slightly better for older children.

Busoni's diagrams give very precise levels of analgesia and provide excellent guidelines for the experienced anaesthetist, whereas for the less skilled, the simpler calculation put forward by Armitage (9,10) may be easier to use. He gives 0.5ml/kg for lumbosacral block, 1ml/kg for thoracolumbar, and 1.25ml/kg for mid-thoracic block. When this calculation gives a volume of less than 20ml, 0.25% bupivacaine is used. For volumes greater than 20ml, one part of water or saline is added to three parts of drug, giving a concentration of 0.19%.

Spiegel used the correlation between spread of analgesia and height, and derived the formula:

$$\text{volume of drug} = 4 \times (D-15)/2$$

where D is the distance from the spine of the seventh cervical vertebra to the sacral hiatus.

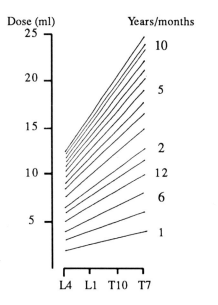

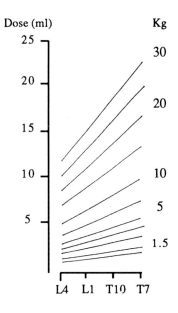

Concentration of local anaesthetic

This influences the type of block produced. For operations such as circumcision, meatotomy, glanduloplasty and superficial surgery of the lower limbs, muscle relaxation is not required, and 1% lidocaine, 1% mepivacaine or 0.25% bupivacaine are sufficient.

If muscle relaxation is needed for the repair of large hernias or for orthopaedic surgery, the concentrations should be increased. Guidance regarding drugs, doses and concentration is given on page 78.

Attempts have been made to utilize the most desirable features of different agents by mixing them together. Seow and Cousins (11) mixed lidocaine and bupivacaine in equal proportions in the hope of combining quick onset of block and muscle relaxation with a long duration of action. The problem of toxicity of such mixtures is discussed in the chapter on pharmacology.

Technique

The child is placed in the lateral position (12,-13,14,15,16) and the legs are flexed. The prone position can be chosen if ketamine was the induction agent or if general anaesthesia is being maintained through an endotracheal tube. Recognition of the anatomical landmarks is easy. The sacro-iliac joints and the sacral hiatus form an equilateral triangle whose apex points inferiorly, and the sacral cornua flank the hiatus (Fig 38). There is considerable anatomical variation in this region.

After identification of the sacral hiatus, the skin is disinfected, and while the skin is drying, two syringes are prepared. One is filled with the test dose and the other with the calculated dose of local anaesthetic.

Fig. 38. Anatomical landmarks in the position of puncture.

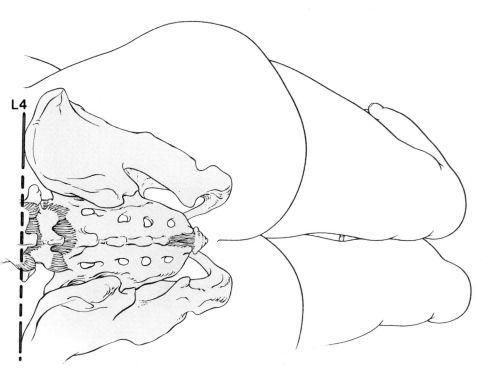

L4

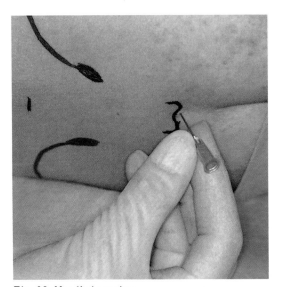

Fig. 39. Needle insertion.

Four points should be observed in the per-formance of a caudal block:

1. the site of needle insertion should first be punctured with a lancet or large bore needle.

2. the caudal needle should be inserted at an angle of 60° to the dorsal surface of the sacrum and directed cephalad (Fig. 39). As it pierces the sacrococcygeal ligament, there is a characteristic, sudden 'give' (Fig. 40) as though the needle had punctured a tight drum skin or membrane. The needle now lies in the epidural space. In Schulte Steinberg's original description of this technique, he suggests that the posterior surface of the anterior table of sacral bone should be located. This is not necessary for the success of the block, but it does ensure that pelvic structures cannot be damaged if this protective bony shield lies between them and the caudal needle.

3. an aspiration test should be performed for blood and CSF, but this is not completely reli-able, and intravascular injection can occur even after a negative test.

Fig. 40. Puncture of the sacral canal.

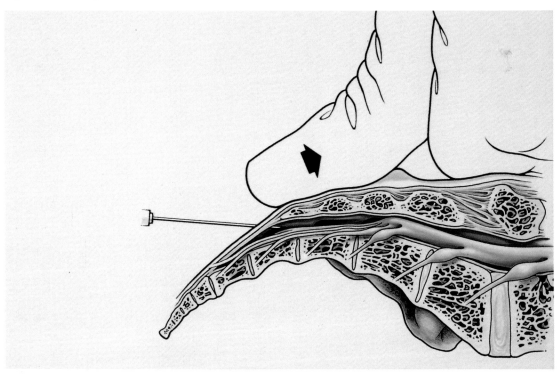

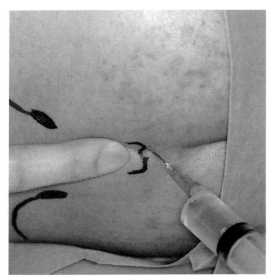

Fig. 41. Injection.

4. a test dose of local anaesthetic, containing adrenaline, should be given to confirm or refute the result of the aspiration test. During the minute following the injection, the ECG is observed for tachycardia or arrhythmia, either of which indicates intravascular placement of the caudal needle. If this test is also negative, the full clinical dose in the second syringe is injected while one or two fingers of the left hand are placed over the dorsum of the sacrum so that an erroneous subcutaneous injection can be recognised early (Figs. 41 and 42). After com-pletion of the injection, the needle is withdrawn and the child positioned for surgery.

In the immediate postoperative period, motor function must be checked in the recovery room and the child should not be returned to the ward until he can move his lower limbs.

Fig. 42. Subcutaneous and intraosseous injections.

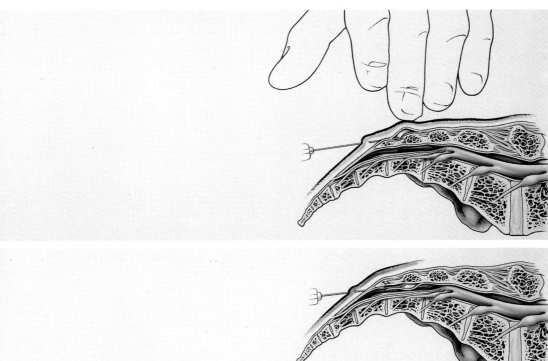

Complications (17)

Subcutaneous injection
Subcutaneous injection on the dorsum of the sacrum. If this is discovered before the full clinical dose has been given, a second attempt may be made, but care must be taken that the toxic dose is not exceeded by the two injections.

Bloody tap
If this occurs, the needle is irrigated and either advanced or withdrawn a short distance. If no blood then appears and the test dose does not produce an intravascular response, the full dose may be given.

Dural puncture
This is very rare indeed if the technique has been correctly performed and no attempt has been made to advance the needle into the sacral canal.

Intravascular and interosseous injection

These should be recognised by the test dose (Fig. 42). Interosseous injection is most likely to occur when needles finer than 20g are used and when contact with the anterior or posterior table of bone is deliberately sought.

Breakage of needle
This is a possible but unlikely complication which can be minimised by previous inspection and testing. Retrieval of a broken needle is facilitated if the needle has not been inserted to its full length.

Perforation of the rectum
This may occur if the needle has been angled too steeply and inserted forcefully in infants. It may also occur if the needle has been accidentally inserted between the sacrum and the coccyx. It is unlikely to happen in experienced hands. If it does occur, the block must be abandoned and the child put on antibiotics and a low residue diet.

Haematoma
This can presumably occur after the puncture of an epidural vein, but is essentially of no consequence.

Sepsis
This is an unlikely complication, but the anaesthetist should always bear the possibility in mind.

Urinary retention
This is extremely rare. A distended bladder can be emptied by gentle suprapubic pressure, and catheterisation is unnecessary.

Conclusion
Caudal block is an easy and safe technique and is suitable for a wide range of surgery in children. It simplifies other aspects of the anaesthetic procedure. For example, it often avoids the need for intubation for short operations, and reduces or eliminates the requirements for muscle relaxants and opioids, with their inherent disadvantages and complications. It allows feeding to start soon after operation, and it provides much better intra-operative analgesia than the inhalational agents alone, without causing adverse haemodynamic changes. If a long- acting local anaesthetic is used, the block will often extend well into the postoperative period, and the technique can be used for day surgery. There is minimal risk of dural puncture if the block is correctly performed.

References
1. Keith I (1977) Anaesthesia and blood loss in total hip replacement. Anaesthesia 32:444
2. Modig J (1982) Thromboembolism and blood loss. Regional Anaesthesia Suppl 7:4,5
3. Chin SP, Abou-Madi M, Eurin B, Witvoet J, Montagne J (1982) Blood loss in total hip replacement. Extradural v. phenoperidine analgesia. Br J Anaesth 54:491
4. McGown RG (1982) Caudal analgesia in children; five hundred cases for procedures below the diaphragm. Anaesthesia 37:806
5. Bromage PR (1975) Mechanism of action of extradural analgesia. British Journal of Anaesthesia 47:199
6. Usubiaga J, Wilkinski J. Usubiaga LE. (1967) Epidural pressure and its relation to spread of anaesthetic solutions in the epidural space. Anesthesia and Analgesia 46:440
7. Schulte Steinberg O, Rahlfs VW (1970) Caudal anaesthesia in children and spread of 1% lignocaine. Br J Anaesth 42:1093

8. Busoni P (1986) The spread of caudal analgesia in children. A mathematical model. Anaesth Intens Care

9. Armitage EN (1979) Caudal block in children. Anaesthesia 34:396

10. Armitage EN (1985) Regional anaesthesia in paediatrics. Clinics in Anaesthesiology 3:555

11. Seow L, Cousins MJ (1982) Lidocaine and bupivacaine mixtures for epidural blockade. Anesthesiology 56:177

12. Cathelin F (1901) Une nouvelle voie d'injection rachidienne, methode des injections epidurales par le procede du canal sacre. Application a l'homme. C.R. Soc Biol 53:452

13. Campbell MJ (1933) Caudal anesthesia in children. American Journal of Urology 3:245

14. Hassan SZ (1977) Caudal anesthesia in infants. Anesth Analg 56:686

15. Soliman MG, Ansara S, Laberge R (1978) Caudal anesthesia in paediatric patients. Canad Anaesth Soc J 25:226

16. Giaufre E, Morisson Lacombe G, Rousset Rouviere B (1983) L'anesthesie caudale en chirurgie pediatrique. Chir pediatr 24:165

17. Massey Dawkins CJ (1969) An analysis of the complications of extradural and caudal block. Anaesthesia 24:554

Continuous caudal block

Paolo Busoni

Continuous caudal anaesthesia (CCA) is an especially interesting technique in children because a catheter passed into the epidural space by the caudal route can reach almost any level. This is due partly to the fact that the epidural fat in children is gelatinous (1) and offers minimal resistance to the passage of a catheter, and partly to the fact that the epidural space itself is said to be very wide and practically empty in newborn and small infants (2). In addition, the progress of a catheter inserted through the sacral hiatus is unlikely to be interrupted, since it runs parallel to the dura. This is almost always true for the newborn and small infants up to about 6kg body weight, and theoretically, any level of epidural anaesthesia - sacral, lumbar, thoracic and even cervical - can be obtained with a continuous caudal technique at a very early age. In older children, catheters are often arrested at L2-3, L3-4 or L4-5 in practice, as will be discussed later.

Fig. 43.The sacral canal.

Indications

Prolonged operations on the limbs, external genitalia, and upper and lower abdomen can be carried out under CCA. Examples include repair of hypospadias and plastic procedures on the male genitalia where a painless postoperative period is particularly desirable, and emergency operations such as intestinal obstruction in the newborn. The author has successfully used the technique in several cases of biliary atresia in which the postoperative course was particularly easy and satisfactory, and Bosenberg et al (2) have also reported success in 20 infants with the same condition. CCA reduces or avoids the need for muscle relaxants, and there is good evidence that this in turn reduces the need for postoperative intensive care as curare-like agents have variable effects in infants and the newborn (3, 4). In addition, the stress response to surgical trauma is said to be reduced in children (5, 6). Research has been limited to children undergoing lower abdominal operations, and no data are available for upper abdominal surgery.

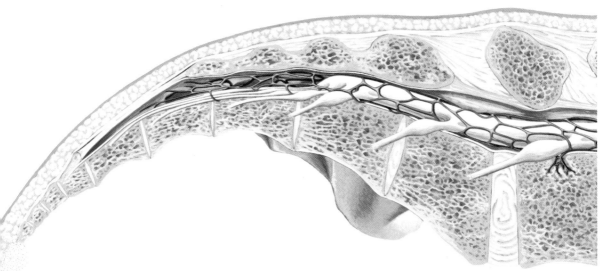

© buckhöj

Advantages

These to some extent overlap with the indications, but may be summarised as follows:

1. muscle relaxants can often be avoided.

2. a comparatively large gauge catheter can be introduced into the epidural space in even the smallest age groups.

3. in the newborn and small infants, the catheter can be passed to almost any level in the epidural space.

4. the technique is easy and can be performed rapidly.

5. the postoperative period is impressively calm. Opiates are unnecessary and the incidence of nausea, vomiting and urinary retention is therefore greatly reduced.

6. intake of oral fluids can commence early in the postoperative period.

7. the necessity for postoperative intensive care is reduced even after the most extensive surgical procedures.

8. effective anaesthesia and analgesia can be produced with small doses of local anaesthetic. In other words, the technique is dose-sparing.

Contraindications

There are no special contraindications

Anaesthetic drugs and dosage

The relationship between dosage, spread of analgesia and age (or body weight and height) is well recognised (7). Bromage (8) studied the effects of 2% lidocaine in patients between the ages of 4 and 18 years, and calculated the mean dose in ml required to anaesthetise one derma-tome. He demonstrated that this dose increases with age, and he derived a formula from which the total volume could be obtained according to the number of analgesic dermatomes required. The author carried out similar research, using 2% mepivacaine (Fig. 44), in 180 cases of CCA in children between one day and 12 years of age. Due to the fact that neonates and small children were included in the study, the resulting interpolating curve was not linear, unlike Bromage's. Both the mean curve and the 90% confidence limits were calculated. A power equation best fits this curve (Fig. 44).

Table. 10. page 90 makes use of both age and weight for calculating the volume of local anaesthetic to inject through the catheter.

Fig. 44. Scatter diagram of the relationship between age and dosage (ml) per spinal segment (2% plain mepivacaine). 90% confidence limits are also shown.

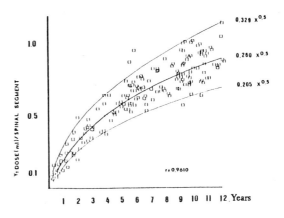

Table 10. Showing the estimated dose (ml) from 3 independent variables (age, weight, upper level of analgesia)

Upper Level	YEARS/Kg	T= 11 (T12)	13 (T10)	16 (T7)	18 (T5)
	60	16.3	17.8	19.8	21.1
	55	16.0	17.5	19.5	20.8
	50	15.8	17.2	19.2	20.4
'12'	45	15.5	16.9	18.9	20.1
	40	15.2	16.6	18.5	19.7
	35	14.9	16.3	18.1	19.3
	30	14.5	15.9	17.7	18.8
	55	15.5	16.9	18.8	20.0
	50	15.2	16.9	18.5	19.7
	45	15.0	16.3	18.2	19.4
'11'	40	14.7	16.0	17.9	19.0
	35	14.4	15.7	17.5	18.6
	30	14.0	15.3	17.0	18.1
	25	13.6	14.8	16.5	17.6
	50	14.6	15.9	17.8	18.9
	45	14.4	15.7	17.5	18.6
	40	14.1	15.4	17.1	18.2
'10'	35	13.8	15.0	16.8	17.8
	30	13.4	14.7	16.3	17.4
	25	13.0	14.2	15.9	16.9
	45	13.7	15.0	16.7	17.0
	40	13.5	14.7	16.4	17.4
'9'	35	13.2	14.4	16.0	17.0
	30	12.8	14.0	15.6	16.6
	25	12.5	13.6	15.2	16.1
	20	12.0	13.1	14.6	15.6
	40	12.8	14.0	15.6	16.6
	35	12.5	13.7	15.2	16.2
'8'	30	12.2	13.3	14.9	15.8
	25	11.8	12.9	14.4	15.3
	20	11.4	12.5	13.9	14.8
	35	11.8	12.9	14.4	15.3
'7'	30	11.5	12.6	14.0	14.9
	25	11.2	12.2	13.6	14.5
	20	10.2	11.8	13.1	14.0

Upper Level	YEARS/Kg	T= 11 (T12)	13 (T10)	16 (T7)	18 (T5)
	30	10.8	11.8	13.1	14.0
	25	10.5	11.4	12.7	13.6
'6'	20	10.1	11.0	12.3	13.1
	15	9.6	10.5	11.7	12.5
	25	9.7	10.6	11.8	12.5
'5'	20	9.3	10.2	11.4	12.1
	15	8.9	9.7	10.8	11.5
	20	8.5	9.3	10.3	11.0
'4'	15	8.1	8.8	9.8	10.5
	10	7.6	8.3	9.2	9.8
	20	7.5	8.2	9.1	9.7
'3'	15	7.2	7.8	8.7	9.3
	10	6.7	7.3	8.1	8.7
'2'	15	6.0	6.6	7.3	7.8
	10	5.6	6.1	6.8	7.3
'1.5'	15	5.3	5.8	6.5	6.9
	10	5.0	5.4	6.0	6.4
months '12'	10.5	4.2	4.6	5.1	5.4
	8.5	4.1	4.4	4.9	5.3
'9'	10.0	3.7	4.0	4.5	4.8
	8.0	3.6	3.9	4.3	4.6
'6'	8.0	3.0	3.3	3.6	3.9
	6.0	2.9	3.1	3.5	3.7
'3'	6.5	2.2	2.4	2.7	2.8
	5.5	2.1	2.3	2.5	2.7
	4.5	2.0	2.2	2.5	2.6
'1'	5.0	1.3	1.4	1.5	1.6
	3.5	1.2	1.3	1.4	1.5
'<1'	4.0	0.92	1.00	1.12	1.19
	3.5	0.90	0.98	1.09	1.18
	2.5	0.85	0.93	1.03	1.10

X=age, W=weight, T=Number of analgesic dermatomes

Model: $Y = aX^{\beta}W^{\gamma}T^{\partial}E$

(E) $Y = 0.817X^{0.430}W^{0.163}T^{0.524}$ estimated dose (ml) 2% Mepivacaine

The catheter technique is dose sparing as the level of analgesia can be tested in the conscious patient. However, in children under general anaesthesia, it is impossible to check the level of analgesia before surgery. When the above table is used, the desired level of analgesia is achieved in 60% of cases. This can be improved to 95% if a slightly larger volume (representing about two additional dermatomes) is injected. If this increased volume is likely to result in a toxic dose being given, the drug can be diluted, as the author's experience has shown that volume is more important than concentration in achieving desired levels of analgesia.

Whenever possible, and if the other forms of anaesthesia being used permit it, the level of analgesia should be checked accurately. Two methods are used. First, the child's response to pin prick is observed. This indicates the level to which the small C fibres have been blocked. Second, severe pinching of the skin is used to test for block of the A delta fibres. This is a very strong stimulus, much resembling surgical stimulation, and the level of block is usually found to be considerably lower than that for pin prick. The reason for testing both of these modalities will be discussed later.

With regard to choice of drug, the author prefers mepivacaine (1%, 1.5% or 2%) because it has been widely used without untoward effects. However, other local anaesthetics can be safely used in equivalent concentration (9,10). The practice of mixing two different anaesthetics has no advantages in CCA and is not recommended, though when profound muscle relaxation is required, etidocaine used in a mixture as 1% or 0.75% gives the best results. It can be injected when needed during surgery. If it is unavailable, 2% lidocaine with adrenaline is an adequate substitute. Adrenaline increases the relaxant effect considerably.

Technique

The child is turned into the lateral position with the legs flexed. An intravenous plastic cannula is inserted through the sacrococcygeal ligament, as described for the single shot technique (7,11). The complete cannula is advanced 1cm into the sacral canal. The metal stylet is then withdrawn and the plastic sheath is advanced an additional 1cm (Fig. 45). This allows the epidural catheter to pass more easily. An epidural catheter of appropriate size is measured against the back of the child from the end of the cannula to the desired spinal level.

The catheter is then inserted through the plastic cannula and carefully and gently advanced (Fig. 46). Usually the catheter can be advanced very easily as far as the lumbar region. In premature babies, infants and small children, the catheter may reach the upper lumbar and even the thoracic regions without meeting any resistance.

Schulte Steinberg studied the results of CCA performed in this way (2). Using radiography and dissection of cadavers, he showed that caudal catheters tend to get caught at the upper lumbar dural cuffs (where spinal nerves leave the epidural space) in older children and those beyond infancy. If catheters were advanced inspite of resistance, the tip was found either to have turned around and run caudally down the epidural canal, or to

Fig. 45. Plastic cannula insertion through the sacrococcygeal ligament.

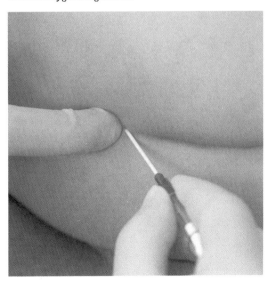

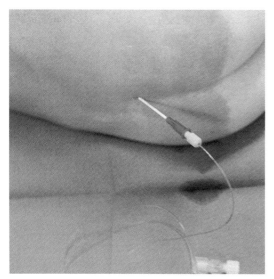

Fig. 46. The catheter is inserted.

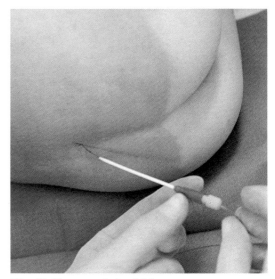

Fig. 47. The cannula is withdrawn

have become lodged at the site of obstruction with the lower end curled up instead. Therefore, if resistance is met, no attempt must be made to advance the catheter, and it should be withdrawn about 1cm. At this stage, manipulation of the child may sometimes dislodge a catheter, which can then be advanced further (2). If after this

manoeuvre, the catheter cannot be passed, the injection of a larger dose of local anaesthetic can compensate for the lack of height and provide anaesthesia to the required level. When the catheter is suitably placed, the cannula is withdrawn (Fig. 47) and the catheter is firmly fixed to the child's back with adhesive tape (Fig. 48).

Fig. 48. The catheter is firmly fixed.

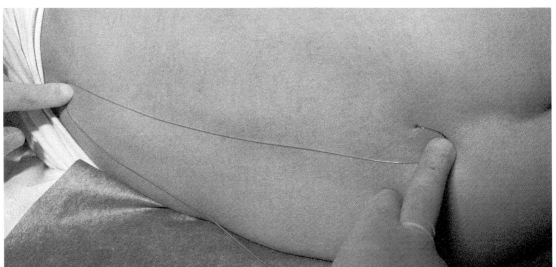

In a study of 30 children between the ages of 1 and 12 years, the author measured the length of catheter in the epidural space, from the tip to the skin puncture site. Fig. 49. shows that in only one case did the catheter reach as high as T6, and usually it was arrested at levels between T12 and L5. However, the X-ray (Fig. 50) shows that, in neonates and small infants, every level can be easily reached, and this is confirmed by studies in cadavers (2). Thus, the height to which a catheter can be threaded in the epidural space depends on the age of the child. An advantage of the caudal route for epidural anaesthesia is that large gauge catheters can be inserted even in the youngest children. In older children, of course, the epidural space can easily be catheterised through the lumbar and thoracic interspaces.

Fig. 50. The catheter has reached as high as T6.

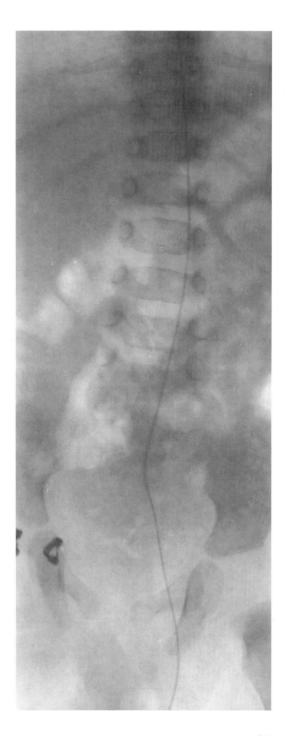

Fig. 49. Scatter diagram of the relationship between age and catheter tip position. Usually catheters arrest between L4-T12.

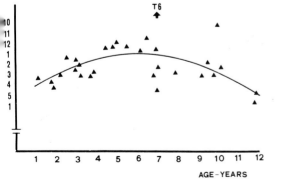

An aspiration test is performed for blood and cerebrospinal fluid and a test dose of an adrenaline-containing solution is given. If no adverse reaction is observed, it is the author's practice to inject one-quarter of the total dose, followed by the remainder after an interval. There must be no resistance to injection. If resistance is felt, it is probably due to kinking or curling of the catheter (Figs. 51 and 52), and the latter should be withdrawn gradually until the resistance disappears.

If the catheter has threaded easily and if there is no resistance to injection, it can be confidently assumed that the catheter is well positioned in the epidural space, that is, without any kink and with the tip facing cephalad. Every effort should be made to achieve this position, as only then will the desired level of anaesthesia be obtained with the minimum volume of local anaesthetic. The size of the catheter should be large enough to allow the drug to be injected at a rate of 0.7ml/sec. If the rate is slower, larger doses of drug will be required to achieve the desired levels of anaesthesia.

Fig. 51. The catheter has curled

Fig. 52. The catheter has kinked

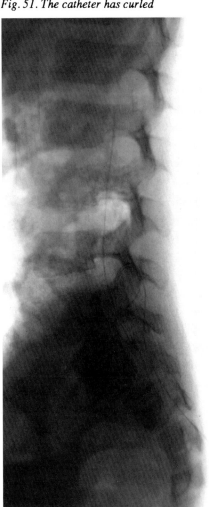

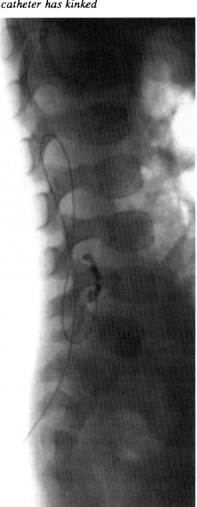

Per-operative management and top-ups

From the time of completion of the local anaesthetic injection (which should be recorded), there follows a very important period of about 15 to 20 minutes during which the child and the attached monitors must be closely observed. The state of the pupils should be noted and they are usually found to be constricted.

If the child is conscious and able to cooperate, his reaction to the stimulus of pin prick and pinching is elicited every five minutes until the upper level of analgesia is clearly established. When 2% mepivacaine is used, the maximum spread of analgesia is reached in 3 to 5 minutes in neonates and infants, while in older children 7 to 10 minutes are needed. As explained earlier, the pinching method indicates the dermatomes devoid of all (even tactile) sensation, whereas only certain modalities are obtunded in the areas analgesic to pin prick.

If the catheter is well positioned with the tip pointing cephalad, the area of analgesia to pin prick is typically at least three dermatomes higher than the area analgesic to pinching. On the other hand, if the catheter is bent, these areas are much closer together and both are lower than expected. These tests can be used (together with easy threading of the catheter and lack of resistance to injection) to confirm the satisfactory positioning of the catheter in the epidural space.

If the breathing of the child is in any way unusual, the pupils must be checked. It should be emphasised that in an anaesthetised or heavily sedated child, the pupils are an excellent indicator of the child's condition. Constricted pupils indicate a satisfactory state with no imminent danger, but if previously constricted pupils start to dilate, this is a warning sign and the anaesthetist must prepare for an emergency. The time is noted and the time interval from completion of the local anaesthetic injection is calculated. There are three possible causes for a change in pupil size:

1. Intravascular injection. This is a possibility if dilatation of the pupil occurs in less than three minutes from the beginning of the procedure and is accompanied by tachycardia (if an adrenaline-containing solution has been used) or bradycardia (if a plain solution has been used).

2. Total spinal due to inadvertent injection into the subarachnoid space. This should be suspected if the pupils are dilated, but unequal, if the pupillary margin is irregular, and if these changes occur after the first three minutes. From the beginning of the procedure there may also be a slight increase in heart rate.

3. Massive absorption of local anaesthetic (perhaps as a result of an overdose). This should be considered when dilatation of the pupils occurs after an interval of more than 10 minutes.

During short operations, the child can be kept calm and quiet with diazepam 0.2mg.kg^{-1} up to a total dose of 10mg. This will not interfere with normal, spontaneous breathing. For operations longer than about 45 minutes, light general anaesthesia can be given by mask. If surgery is likely to be very prolonged and tedious, the author favours balanced anaesthesia with nasotracheal intubation. Nasotracheal intubation is well tolerated by children, and breathing can be assisted by synchronised intermittent mandatory ventilation (SIMV) - an excellent method of assistance - or by hand. In the youngest children, fully controlled ventilation is preferred. This is easily accomplished if the block is successful and the level of analgesia is adequate.

When 2% mepivacaine is used, top-up injections are required soon after the first hour, when half of the initial dose can be given and repeated hourly. Supplementary analgesic drugs are not usually necessary.

In most cases the catheter is removed at the end of surgery because of the danger of infection from soiling. A dose of bupivacaine, in the same volume as the intraoperative top-ups, may be given just prior to removal.

Children are very sensitive to the acute pain which is present for the first few hours after surgery (12,13,14). Pain in the later postoperative period is usually well tolerated and, in the author's experience, the final top-up, given just before removal of the catheter, is sufficient in the majority of cases and further supplementary analgesics are unnecessary.

Complications

In over 1.000 cases, the author has encountered no serious complications at any time. The incidence of vomiting in the first 24 hours was 5%. This mainly occurred several hours after operation when the expulsive reflexes were fully active and the danger of aspiration was therefore minimal.

The lack of serious complications in this series can be explained in part by the fact that only fully trained, experienced anaesthetists were performing CCA. However, all the complications described in adult patients can presumably also occur in children, and since the catheter is threaded a considerable distance up the epidural space, damage to the thin walled vessels of the venous plexus, with subsequent bleeding, is an obvious possible hazard.

Schulte Steinberg et al. carried out some experiments to elucidate this. They introduced caudal epidural catheters into anaesthetised piglets and threaded the catheters to very high levels. If resistance occurred, the catheters were deliberately and forcefully advanced further. Ten minutes later, the animals were sacrificed by bleeding, and the epidural canal was subsequently dissected for evidence of haemorrhage and gross neural damage. No trace of either was found, and this was true even where the catheter had been forcefully advanced. In these cases, the catheter was found either to have doubled back on itself or to have curled up from below. One important message emerges from these studies. It is useless to expect that a catheter tip can be forced past an obstruction, if this cannot be overcome by manipulation, and no attempt should be made to do this. However, the studies also do appear to indicate that the technique is safe and, in particular, that epidural haematomas do not seem to be produced, even when the catheter is advanced to thoracic levels or when it doubles back or curls up. It is of course obvious, as stated earlier in this chapter, that CCA should only be used in children in whom the coagulation tests are normal.

Clotted blood was found occluding the catheter in 3% of cases. It has to be washed out with saline, and the previously- described tests accurately carried out to ensure that the catheter does not lie in a blood vessel - lowering the catheter hub below the patient to observe any flow-back of blood, and giving an adrenaline-containing injection down the catheter to elicit a cardio-vascular response.

Although the sacral hiatus appears to be relatively high due to the peculiarities of the infant's anatomy, it is in fact near to the anus, and soiling is a risk. It seems wise, therefore, to remove the catheter at the end of the operation. Cultures taken from catheters after removal have failed to grow any pathogens.

Conclusions

CCA is a safe and easy technique with many advantages. However, it is evident that:

1. Children must be selected carefully. Preoperative evaluation must be thorough, and coagulopathies and dehydration must be corrected.

2. The anaesthetist must be experienced and fully trained in regional block technique in children.

3. Close monitoring of the pupils, heart rate, blood pressure and respiration is essential.

CCA provides excellent access to the higher levels of the epidural space particularly in prematures, neonates and young infants. It is a simpler and easier alternative to the more delicate direct lumbar and thoracic approaches. The usefulness becomes very obvious in the neonate in whom the neuromuscular junction is immature and in whom the anaesthetist may prefer to avoid muscle relaxants and the possible need for post operative ventilation.

References

1. Tretjakoff D (1926) Das Epidurale Fettgewebe. Z Anat 79:100
2. Bosenberg AT, Bland BAR, Schulte Steinberg O, Downing JW (1988) Thoracic epidural anaesthesia via the caudal route in infants and children. Anesthesiology 69:265
3. Crumrine RS, Yodlowski EH (1981) Assessment of neuromuscular function in infants. Anesthesiology 54:29
4. Fisher DM, O'Keefe C, Stanski DR, Cronnely R, Miller RD, Gregory GA (1982) Pharmacokinetics and pharmacodynamics of d-tubocurarine in infants, children and adults. Anesthesiology 57:203
5. Boninsegni R, Salerno R, Giannotti P, Andreuccetti T, Busoni P, Santoro S, Forti G (1983) Effects of surgery and epidural or general

anaesthesia on testosterone, 17-hydroxyprogesterone and cortisol plasma levels in prepubertal boys. J.Steroid Biochem 19:1783

6. Giaufre E, Conte-Devolx B, Morisson-Lacombe G, Boudouresque F, Grino M, Rousset-Pouviere B, Guilame V, Oliver C (1985) Anesthesie peridurale par voie caudale chez l'enfant: etude des variations endocriniennes. La presse medicale 14 N.4:201

7. Schulte Steinberg O, Rahlfs VW (1970) Caudal anaesthesia in children and spread of 1% lignocaine: a statistical study. Brit J Anaesth 42:1093

8. Bromage PR (1969) Ageing and epidural dose requirements: segmental spread and predictability of epidural analgesia in youth and extreme age. Brit J Anaesth 41:1016

9. Schulte Steinberg O, Rahlfs VW (1977) Spread of extradural analgesia following caudal injection in children. A statistical study. Brit J Anaesth 49:1027

10. Andreuccetti T, Busoni P, Romiti M (1983) Diffusione dell'analgesia epidurale sacrale di tre anestetici locali (lidocaina 2%, mepivacaina 2%, bupivacaina 0.5%): studio statistico su 418 pazienti in eta'pediatrica. Anest Rianim 24:95

11. Busoni P, Andreuccetti T, Romiti M (1981) Diffusione dela mepivacaina dopo blocco epidurale sacrale in pediatrica. Studio statistico. Anest Rianim 22:67

12. Owens ME (1984) Pain in infancy: conceptual and methodological issues. Pain 20:213

13. Savedra M, Gibbons P, Tesler M, Ward J, Wegner C (1982) How do children describe pain? A tentative assessment. Pain 14:95

14. Levine JD, Gordon NC (1982) Pain in prelingual children and its evolution by pain-induced vocalisation. Pain 14:85

Single shot lumbar epidural block

Elisabeth Giaufre

Elisabeth Giaufre

Fig. 53. Single shot lumbar epidural block

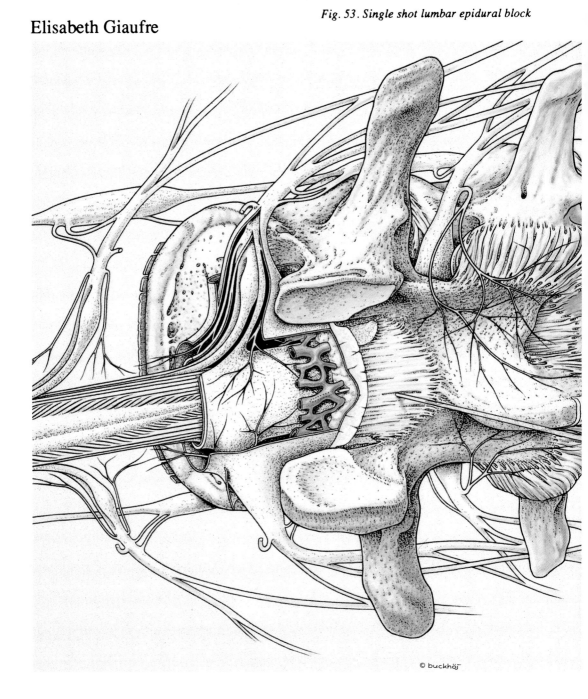

© buckhöj

Low lumbar and caudal epidural blocks are the most commonly used central blocks because the needle is inserted caudad to the termination of the spinal cord, and the risk of damage to it is therefore small.

Indications

This form of epidural block is suitable for operations lasting less than about 90 minutes, involving dermatomes between T5 and S5 and for which postoperative epidural analgesia is unnecessary. Examples include the repair of umbilical hernia, appendicitis, intussusception, reimplantation of ureters and surgery for intraabdominal testis.

Contraindications

These are the same as for the single shot caudal technique. The method is unsuitable for procedures which are likely to outlast the duration of the block, and for upper abdominal surgery, where a thoracic block is to be preferred. It is also unsuitable if previous surgery has been performed at or near the epidural puncture site, as for the insertion of Harrington rods or CD (Cotrel-Dubousset) material, for example.

Choice of drugs

Dose requirements

Busoni (1), using statistical methods, found that although the level of analgesia is very predictable after caudal block, it can only be approximately predicted after lumbar epidural block. This is clearly demonstrated when Figures 54 and 55 are compared. The former illustrates the situation for caudal block and the latter for lumbar. The difference may lie in the fact that solution injected through the sacral hiatus can only spread upwards, whereas solution injected by the lumbar route can spread both up and down, thus making the result more variable.

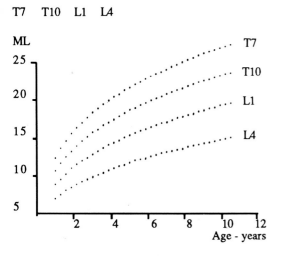

Fig. 54. Level of analgesia correlated to age and volume, caudal block (P Busoni).

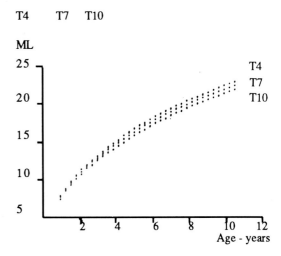

Fig. 55. Level of analgesia correlated to age and volume, lumbar block (P Busoni).

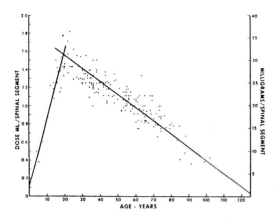

Fig. 56. Relationship of extradural dose requirements to age (2% lignocaine supine). (From Bromage PR (1969) Ageing and epidural dose requirements. Br J Anaesth 41:1016.

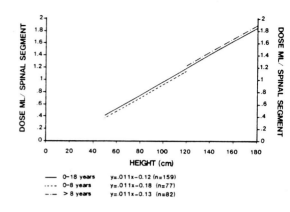

Fig. 57. Dose related to height. I Murat personal data

Three formulae have been suggested for calculation of the dose. Bromage (2) (Fig 56) used 2% lidocaine, but this is not suitable for children under 4 years of age. Busoni's regime, illustrated in his diagram (Table 10, page 90), uses 2% mepivacaine and is widely used in current anaesthetic practice. A third formula uses 0.25% bupivacaine in a dose of 0.75ml.kg^{-1} for children under the age of 8 years or weighing less than 25kg and 1ml.kg^{-1} for every 10cm of height for older children (3.4). These dosages provide blocks of 10 to 12 segments (Figs. 57 and 58).

Concentration

For intra-abdominal surgery, a significant degree of motor block is required and this can be obtained by using higher concentrations of local anaesthetic, such as 2% lidocaine, 0.5% bupivacaine and 2% mepivacaine with adrenaline.

Fig. 58. Dose related to weight.I Murat personal data

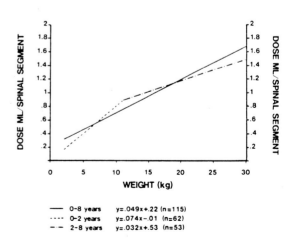

Technique

A reliable intravenous line is first established, and the lumbar epidural injection is performed with the child sedated or under general anaesthesia. For the single shot, the paramedian approach is not recommended unless abnormal anatomical landmarks are encountered, as the sedated or anaesthetised child cannot give warning if a complication arises. Children usually have perfect landmarks, the epidural space is most easily identified at the L2-L3 level, and the midline approach, being easier technically, is preferred (Fig. 59).

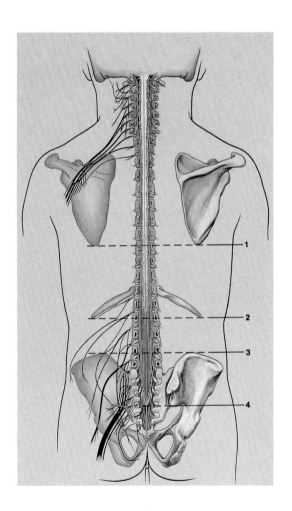

Fig. 59. Anatomical landmarks for lumbar single shot.

1. Inferior angle of scapulae (Spinous process of T7)
2. Rib margin (L2)
3. Superior aspect of iliac crest (L4)
4. Posterior superior iliac spine (S3)

Midline lumbar epidural puncture

The iliac crests and the spine of L4 are identified (Fig 60) and a wide area of surrounding skin is cleaned with antiseptic solution. Two syringes are prepared, one containing the test dose, and the other the clinical dose. The distance between the skin and the epidural space can be estimated, as there is a strong correlation between this distance and age. Busoni has shown that, at the L2-3 interspace, the distance in mm is 10 + (age in years x 2). Kosaka (5) has derived a formula for the distance at the L3-4 interspace. These formulae are useful guides.

There are four stages in the performance of lumbar epidural puncture.

From skin to ligamentum flavum

The thumb of the left hand, pressed perpendicular to the skin, marks the midline at the upper part of the chosen space. Alternatively, this area can be defined by straddling the midline with two fingers of the left hand. The Tuohy needle is advanced in the midline, with the right hand, at an angle of 90° in the newborn and 70° in children (Fig. 60). During insertion, the bevel of the needle should face laterally to separate rather than cut the longitudinally running fibres of the ligaments and, in case of an accidental puncture, the dura (Fig. 61). When the needle has engaged in the ligament, it should feel like an arrow in a target.

Fig. 60. Needle position while piercing the skin.

Fig. 61. Child's spine in the position of puncture.

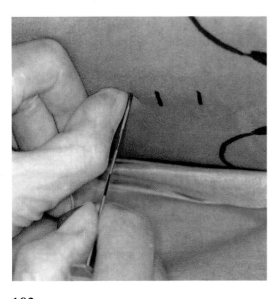

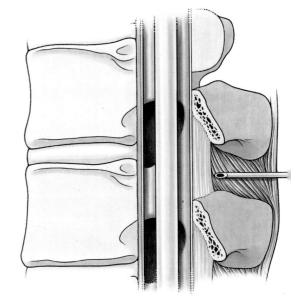

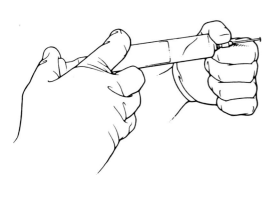

Fig. 62. "Bromage" grip.

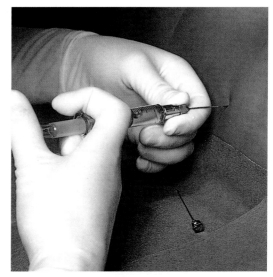

Fig. 63. Modified grip resulting from the shortness of some paediatric needles.

From ligament to epidural space

The stylet is removed and the syringe to be used for identification of the epidural space is locked onto the needle. The needle is then firmly held, at the junction of the hub and shaft so that the grip exerts a three-point fixation, with the metacarpal heads braced against the patient's back. This is known as Bromage's grip (Figs. 62):

"The hand is supinated, with the wrist partially flexed and the back of the carpus braced against the patient´s back. Forward motion is imparted to the needle by a gradual extension of the wrist, and the carpus and metacarpus roll in toward the back like an eccentric cam driving piston." (Ph Bromage)

As soon as the ligamentum flavum is pierced, resistance to the syringe plunger is lost and the needle is immediately halted.

The syringe is removed and care is taken not to move the needle.

Thus, the epidural space has been identified by loss of resistance (Fig. 64). Only a small volume of air or saline should be used, 0.5ml being sufficient in the neonate, and 3ml being the maximum in older children, so that when the local anaesthetic solution is injected, its spread or concentration are not affected.

Macintosh's balloon is little used for locating the epidural space in children because the softness of the tissues may allow it to deflate before the space has been reached. If fluid appears from the needle when the stylet is removed, cerebrospinal fluid can be distinguished from local anaesthetic or saline solution by the fact that it is at body temperature, and the dextrostix test will give a positive reaction for sugar (8). Furthermore, a dural tap produces a continuous drip from the

Fig. 64. The epidural space has been identified by loss of resistance.

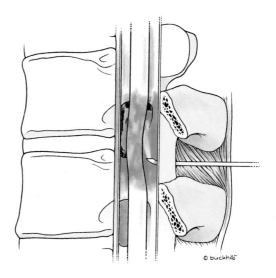

103

needle whereas flow of injected fluid tends to slow down and will eventually stop.

In children of less than 4 kg, a 23 g Butterfly needle may be used instead of the Tuohy. The technique is the same as far as the ligamentum flavum, but thereafter, the left hand alone advances the needle by gripping the wings of the needle between thumb and forefinger, with the wrist resting on table or trolley. A syringe is connected to the Butterfly tubing and the right thumb pushes gently on the plunger to locate the epidural space. When local anaesthetic is injected, it should be remembered that the dead space of the tubing is 0.2ml.

Aspiration test
This should always be performed before injection of local anaesthetic solution even if there is no evidence of dural or vascular tap.

Injection of local anaesthetic
The test dose - of local anaesthetic with adrenaline - is given first, followed by the remaining dose if no reaction to the test dose has been noted. With both Tuohy and Butterfly needles, the injection must be made at low pressure for safety reasons. As there will be a positive pressure in the epidural space at the end of the injection, the needle should be left in place for a few seconds to avoid escape of some solution along the needle track. When the needle has been removed, the child is positioned for surgery.

The author believes that the spread of solution within the epidural space can be extended if the intra-abdominal pressure is increased. Although this has not been verified in controlled trials and must therefore be regarded as anecdotal, particular attention should nevertheless be paid to the level of the block in cases where the position of the patient, or any other factors, may produce a high intra-abdominal pressure.

After operation, the extent of the block should be assessed, and motor block should have worn off before the child is returned to the ward.

Complications (9)
All the complications of a single shot procedure may occur where the full clinical dose has to be injected as a bolus rather than as increments.

Total spinal block
This is easily identified. The first sign is a change in the respiratory rate. There is not necessarily any fall in blood pressure, contrary to the situation in adults. The pupils first become unequal, then dilated, and apnoea eventually follows. The child must be intubated and mechanically ventilated with 100% oxygen until the effects of the total spinal have worn off. This may take 30 minutes to 2 hours, depending on the dose and the agent used. If the situation is under control, there is no reason to postpone surgery.

Misplaced injection
If the loss of resistance sign has been indefinite or misleading, it is possible for the injection to be made superficial to the epidural space. If this occurs, segmental anaesthesia will not be obtained.

Dural puncture
This is not in itself dangerous as long as the anaesthetist recognises that it has occurred. If he fails to realise what has happened and accidentally injects the epidural dose intrathecally, a total spinal will result. The epidural procedure may be attempted at another interspace, but great care must be taken to ensure that total spinal anaesthesia does not occur due to passage of the local anaesthetic into the CSF through the dural perforation (10). Dural puncture may well result in a headache, but it can be treated with an epidural blood patch. There is much to be said in favour of doing this as soon as the error has been noticed so that the child is not subjected to a separate procedure at a later date. The child's own blood is injected epidurally and the volume of blood should be half that of the local anaesthetic dose.

Unilateral or patchy block

This is unusual after a single shot injection, but it can occur due to uneven spread of local anaesthetic. Very occasionally, the epidural space contains fibrous septa which form anatomical barriers and prevent even spread.

Hypotension

Serious hypotension is rare in infants (4), but is a warning sign of other complications, and all other vital signs must be checked. The treatment is the same as for adults.

Vascular puncture

The block can be repeated at another interspace. Although this has been criticised in the past, it is now regarded as acceptable practice in infants and children.

Conclusion

Single shot lumbar epidural block is an easy, safe and useful technique for the many short paediatric operations which involve the lower thoracic and lumbar dermatomes, and which do not require epidural analgesia postoperatively. However, it has not achieved the same popularity in children as in adults, and this may well be due to the fact that suitable equipment has not been available. The situation has improved recently, and paediatric needles and catheters are now obtainable.

References

1. Busoni P (1982) Lumbar extradural anaesthesia in newborn infants and children. ESRA meeting, Edinburgh
2. Bromage PR (1969) Ageing and epidural dose requirements. Brit.J.Anaesth. 41:1016
3. Delleur MM, Murat I, Esteve C, Raynaud P, Gadiche O, Saint Maurice C (1985) Anesthesie peridurale continue chez l'enfant de moins de deux ans. Ann.Fr.Anesth.Reanim. 4:413
4. Murat I, Delleur MM, Esteve C, Egu JF Raynaud P, Saint-Maurice C (1987) Continuous epidural anaesthesia in children: clinical and haemodynamic implications. Br J Anaesth 59:1441
5. Kosaka Y, Sato I, Kawaguchi R (1974) Distance from skin to epidural space in children. Jpn J Anesthesiol 23:874
6. Macintosh R (1978) Lumbar puncture and spinal analgesia. Longman Group Ltd. Churchill Livingstone
7. Haberer J (1980) Anesthesie peridurale. Precis anesthesie loco- regionnale. Gautier Lafaye Edit Masson 180
8. Cousins MJ (1980) Epidural neural blockade. Philadelphia. Lippincott
9. Massey Dawkins CJ (1969) An analysis of the complications of extradural and caudal blocks. Anaesthesia 24:554
10. Bromage PR (1985) Complications of regional anesthesia. ASA Annual Refresher Course lecture 255

Continuous lumbar epidural block

Marie Madeleine Delleur

Introduction

Continuous epidural anaesthesia is of great interest for major surgical procedures in children because it provides really effective post-operative analgesia. It also reduces the amount of systemic analgesics and muscle relaxants required during operation, and there is therefore less risk of residual ventilatory depression in the post-operative period.

Special equipment suitable for use in children is now available, so epidural block can easily be performed even in the youngest patients. It is essential, however, that the anaesthetist is fully trained in epidural technique in adults before he performs it in children.

Indications

1. Any major procedure involving the dermatomes from T5 to S5 is suitable for epidural block.

2. Major surgery of long duration, that is, lasting more than 1 hour, may also qualify and may include abdominal procedures such as the pull-through operation for Hirschsprung's disease (1, 2, 3), various orthopaedic operations such as the correction of club foot and the insertion of prostheses, and genito-urinary operations ranging from reconstructive renal procedures to complex hypospadias repairs and plastic surgery of the external genitalia.

3. Children with pulmonary and muscle diseases benefit from epidural block because it provides a safe recovery phase even after prolonged surgery and gives complete pain control without causing ventilatory depression.

4. Epidural analgesia should be considered for any operation which results in severe post-operative pain and which requires early physiotherapy and painful nursing procedures.

Contraindications

These are the same as for the single-shot technique.

Drug and dosage

Choice of drug

When a continuous technique is to be used, it is important that accumulation of the local anaesthetic drug is minimal, and long-lasting agents should therefore be chosen (4).

Initial dose

The initial dose depends on the height and weight of the child, and on the local anaesthetic used. The concentration chosen will depend on the surgical procedure and on whether muscle relaxation is required.

Technique

The equipment and materials required are discussed in the appropriate chapter.

General anaesthesia

General anaesthesia with endotracheal intubation and controlled ventilation is almost always used.

Lumbar epidural puncture

See also single-shot epidural chapter.

The child is placed in the lateral position. An interspinous space between L3-L4 and T12-L1 is selected, depending on the surgical procedure. At the former level, the risk of damage to the spinal cord is low because the cord usually terminates at or above this point. However, epidural puncture and insertion of a catheter at T12-L1, or higher in the thoracic region, does carry some risk and general anaesthesia is contraindicated except for some very unusual circumstances, so that the patient can monitor a needle by his reaction if it approaches the spinal cord.

A Tuohy needle should be selected appropriate to the size of the child. For those between 1 and 4 years, 20G or 19G needles are suitable. They accept catheters with an external diameter between 0.5 and 0.8mm with or without a stylet. For children over 4 years, 19G or 18G needles may be used. They accept catheters with an external diameter between 0.7 and 1mm with or without mandrin. The anaesthetist must check that the catheter fits the needle before he embarks on the epidural puncture.

The median approach is recommended, with identification of the epidural space by loss of resistance to injection. When the space has been located, the catheter is inserted. Some resistance is often felt when it reaches the tip of the needle. If the catheter contains a stylet, it must now be removed so that the end of the catheter is free, soft and atraumatic. The function of the stylet is to maintain the rigidity of the catheter as it passes through the needle - it must never be allowed to enter the epidural space.

The length of the catheter relative to the needle must be known and not more than 2 or 3 cm should be inserted into the epidural space (Figs. 65 and 66), otherwise the catheter may change direction, pass through an intervertebral foramen or become knotted. When the catheter has been inserted, the needle is very slowly withdrawn so that the catheter is not pulled out with it or transected by the directional bevel. The catheter's position can be verified by reference to the graduation marks along its length, and it can be partially withdrawn if necessary.

When the catheter is being fixed care must be taken to prevent it being kinked or dislodged. A transparent surgical dressing such as OpSite is ideal because any blood in the catheter or infec-

Fig. 65. The catheter should be inserted 2 or 3 cm into the epidural space.

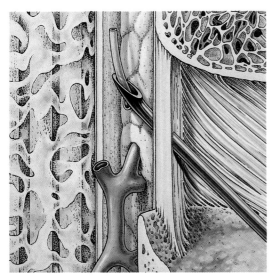

Fig. 66. The catheter in the epidural space.

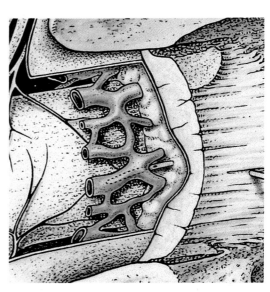

tion at the puncture site can be instantly seen.

Every precaution must be taken against contamination. Full aseptic technique must be maintained throughout the entire procedure and a microbacterial filter, capable of excluding particles larger than 0.22μ, should be used for each injection (6).

Before each injection, an aspiration test must be carried out to ensure that no blood or cerebrospinal fluid enters the catheter. Since a negative aspiration test does not completely exclude intravenous placement of the catheter, a test dose of 1 to 2ml of local anaesthetic with adrenaline 1 in 200.000 is given.

Epidural catheters are useful for postoperative analgesia, and they are well tolerated. They should generally be removed after 72 hours unless there are compelling clinical reasons for keeping them in longer. The risks of the catheter becoming infected (6) and its tip migrating into either a blood vessel or the cerebrospinal fluid increase after this time. In practice, conventional analgesics give adequate results after the third postoperative day in most cases (see chapter on postoperative analgesia).

Advantages

During surgery, opioids and muscle relaxants are required either in reduced dosage or not at all, with a consequent lack of respiratory depression extending into the early postoperative period.

Very few satisfactory studies of the haemodynamic effects of epidural block in children are available, but workers in this field are in general agreement that minimal haemodynamic changes occur. This is certainly true for caudal block (7) and for children aged less than 2 in whom epidural block was induced with 0.25% bupivacaine with adrenaline (5). A recent study by the present authors (9) confirmed that this was also the case in children under 8 years old when epidural anaesthesia was combined with general anaesthesia and when top-ups were given by bolus injection. Pre-loading with intravenous fluids was found to be unnecessary. The changes observed in older children are similar to those found in adults (see chapter on physiology).

Top-up injections, given through an epidural catheter, can be used to provide anaesthesia for prolonged surgery and analgesia postoperatively. The pharmacokinetics of single-shot epidural anaesthesia are well known in children (p. 54), but when a continuous epidural block or repeated top-ups are being given, the risk of accumulation and toxicity should be considered, especially in the postoperative period (10).

In children, plasma levels of bupivacaine ranged between 0.40 and 1.13 μg/ml (mean 0.85 +- 0.10μg/ml) after the first repeat injection of bupivacaine 0.25% with adrenaline (Fig. 67).

These values were about 20% higher than those obtained after the first injection (0.71+- 0.10 μg/ml). This increase can be explained by the elimination half-life calculated after the first injection (227 +- 37.7 min). The pharmacokinetic parameters of bupivacaine obtained after the first repeat injection were unchanged (11).

Fig. 67. Plasma levels of bupivacaine in children 1-7 years of age (11).

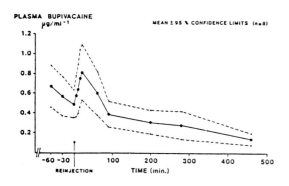

PLASMA BUPIVACAINE
μg/ml⁻¹

MEAN ± 95 % CONFIDENCE LIMITS (n=8)

Complications

All the complications listed for single-shot epidural block apply also to the continuous technique, but there are, of course, additional ones arising from the use of a catheter. Insertion of the catheter may damage a blood vessel and produce a haematoma (10). At a later stage, the tip may become dislodged and may enter a blood vessel or puncture the dura, giving rise, respectively, to the possibility of intravascular and intrathecal injection. An indwelling catheter, like all foreign bodies, is liable to become infected if left in place for a long time.

Complications may also arise from the effects of an epidural block acting continuously over a period of days. Haemodynamic changes after top-ups are minimal. Urinary retention is unusual, but many of the operations for which continuous epidural anaesthesia is indicated require a urinary catheter in the postoperative period so the problem of retention does not arise. Accumulation of local anaesthetic, resulting in rising plasma concentrations, has been described in adults who have been receiving continuous infusions for many hours (12), but not in those receiving intermittent top-ups. No comparable study is available for children.

No complications have been reported in children, and none has been observed by the author.

Summary

Continuous lumbar epidural anaesthesia is of interest in children as a means of producing anaesthesia for operations of long duration. Since opioids can be avoided, the technique allows a rapid and safe recovery. The quality of postoperative analgesia is excellent.

There is a wide margin of safety when bupivacaine with adrenaline is given in the recommended dosage, and this applies both to the initial injection and to subsequent top-ups.

References

1. Ruston FG (1964) Epidural anesthesia in pediatric surgery: present status in the Hamilton General Hospital. Can Anaesth Soc J 11
2. Ruston FG (1954) Epidural anesthesia in infants and children. Can Anaesth Soc J 1:37
3. Ruston FG (1957) Epidural anesthesia in pediatric surgery. Anesth Analg (Cleve) 36:76
4. Tucker GT, Mather LE (1975) Pharmacokinetics of local anaesthetic agents. Br J Anaesth 47:213
5. Delleur MM, Murat I, Esteve C, Raynaud P, Gaudiche O, Saint-Maurice C (1985) Anesthesie peridurale continue chez l'enfant demoins de deux ans. Ann Fr Anesth Reanim 4:413
6. Bromage PR (1978) Epidural analgesia. Philadelphia Saunders. Drugs and equipment
7. Melman E, Pennelas J, Maruffo J (1975) Regional anesthesia in children. Anesth Analg (Cleve) 54:387
8. Fortuna A (1967) Caudal analgesia: a simple and safe technique in paediatric surgery. Br J Anaesth 39:165
9. Murat I, Delleur MM, Esteve C, Egu JF, Raynaud P, Saint-Maurice C (1987) Continuous epidural anaesthesia in children: clinical and haemodynamic implications. Br J Anaesth 59:1441
10. Lienhart A (1986) Les accidents des rachianesthésies et des anesthésies péridurales utilisant les anesthésiques locaux. Anesthésie loco-régionale JEPU- Arnette
11. Murat I, Montay G, Delleur MM, Esteve C et Saint-Maurice C (1988) Bupivacaine pharmacokinetics during epidural anaesthesia in children. Eur J Anaesth 5:113
12. Richter O, Klein K, Abel J, Ohnesorge FK, Wüst HJ, Thussen MM (1984) The kinetics of bupivacaine plasma concentrations during epidural anaesthesia following intra-operative bolus injection and subsequent continuous infusion. International Journal of Clinical Pharmacology, Therapy and Toxicology 22,11:611

Single shot thoracic epidural block

Paolo Busoni

Introduction

Due to the conciderable risk involved in performing thoracic epidural block in the **unconscious** child, this technique should only be used in exceptional circumstances and it should only be performed by an anaesthetist who is experienced in the practice of regional anaesthesia. Written, informed consent should be optained from the parents and inserted in the records of the child, and the surgeon should also be informed.

Indications

The disadvantage of lumbar and caudal epidural blocks is that a large volume of solution has to be injected if midthoracic block is required, and there is then an increased risk of systemic toxicity. Moreover, block of the lumbar and sacral nerves, which is necessarily associated with these techniques, has some specific dis-advantages in the postoperative period, such as residual motor weakness and urinary retention. Thoracic epidural anaesthesia (TEA) avoids these problems. The main indication for thoracic epidural analgesia (TEA) in children is for upper abdominal surgery. The choice between the single shot and the catheter technique largely depends upon the estimated duration of surgery and the need for postoperative pain relief. Although a single dose of local anaesthetic may outlast the surgical procedure and may therefore contribute to analgesia in the immediate postoperative period, it is obvious that a catheter in the epidural space can provide better controlled and longer lasting analgesia.

TEA provides excellent operating conditions, often avoids the need for muscle relaxant drugs, and is safe. It also reduces the time for which postoperative intensive care is needed.

It should be done with the patient awake. General anaesthesia is to be avoided so that the patient can monitor the advancing needle by his reaction. Only in very rare, unusual situations, where a thoracic epidural block cannot be replaced by a less precarious method and where the performance without general anaesthesia is impossible it may be considered.

Contraindications

Abnormalities of the vertebrae are a relative contraindication because underlying structures and anatomical relationships may also be abnormal. Deformity of the bony spine is not actually a contraindication, but it renders the technique much more difficult and therefore more hazardous. However, if the block can be safely performed in such cases, the post-operative rewards are considerable because any associated respiratory disability is minimised.

Drugs and dosage

The dose is calculated, and the concentration selected, on a weight basis. For children of less than 10kg, 1% mepivacaine or 1% lidocaine is used, and the volume given (in ml) is one-third of the body weight in kg. When the weight exceeds 10kg, 1 or 2% mepivacaine or lidocaine is used, and the volume given (in ml) is one-quarter of the body weight in kg.

With this regime, analgesia spreads from T2-3 to T12. Increasing this dose is not advisable as it may produce unwanted analgesia, spreading up to the T1 distribution on the inside of the upper arm, and downwards to the lumbar and sacral dermatomes, affecting the legs. It is important to remember that, on the chest wall, the skin above the T2 dermatome is supplied by C4. It is therefore impossible to obtain analgesia in this area without the risk of gross overdosage, and the anaesthetist must be certain that the operation will not encroach into this region.

Additional drugs

It is obviously necessary to keep the child calm and quiet during surgery, so it is wise to continue with light general anaesthesia or to give intravenous diazepam in a dose of 0.1-.0.2mg.kg^{-1} up to a maximum of 10mg. Similar benzo-diazepines may be given in equipotent doses. If surgery is likely to exceed 30-45 minutes, it is advisable to intubate and ventilate the child.

Technique

Epidural puncture can be performed at any thoracic interspace, but the following description refers to the midthoracic region at T6-7 as this is located near the centre of those dermatomes which need to be blocked for upper abdominal surgery. An injection at this level will therefore provide an effective block with a comparatively small dose of local anaesthetic (1). Another reason for selecting this level is that it highlights the technical difficulties which can occur with the thoracic approach, since the angulation required of the epidural needle is at its greatest in the midthoracic region. Above and below this level, the angulation decreases until, at the lower thoracic interspaces, the needle is inserted perpendicular to the child's back.

The child is placed in the left lateral position with the legs flexed. The angles of the scapulae are identified. The line joining them crosses the vertebral column at the 7th interspace (2).

Either the midline or the paramedian approach can be used. In adults, the paramedian approach is often preferred, but in children, the midline approach is easy and successful and it was used in 95% of the author's cases. In the remaining 5%, it was impossible to reach the epidural space from the midline and the paramedian route had to be used instead.

Fig. 69. The needle is gripped with both hands and a Macintosh ballon is used to find the epidural

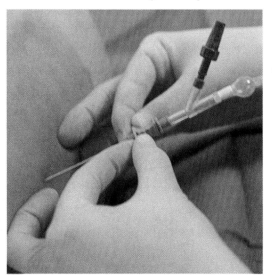

Midline approach

The spinous process of T7 is identified and an indentation is made with the thumb nail in the middle of the T6-7 interspace. The skin is cleaned with antiseptic solution and carefully draped.

The skin in the centre of the interspace should first be incised with a small lancet or large bore needle to prevent carriage of an epidermal plug into the deeper tissues. The epidural needle is then inserted at this site, with a cephalad angulation of 70° to the long axis of the spine. A thin-walled, 19G Crawford or Tuohy needle is used for children over 2 years. For those younger, an ordinary 23G "Butterfly" may be used. The extension tubing is useful in providing greater flexibility to the whole system. There is continuous resistance as the needle passes through the supraspinous and interspinous ligaments, until, in children over one year of age, the characteristic resistance of the liga-mentum flavum is noted. In the youngest children, however, the resistance of the ligamentum flavum is not noticeably different from the more superficial ligaments.

The "loss of resistance" test to identify the epidural space is performed with a 5ml syringe containing 2-3ml normal saline. The Macintosh balloon may also be used, and as it allows the needle to be gripped with both hands (Fig. 69), it is preferred by many anaesthetists.

However, the entire bevel of the needle must be embedded in the ligament before the balloon is attached, otherwise the air tends to escape into the softer, surrounding tissues and the balloon will not remain inflated.

Some anaesthetists prefer air to normal saline for identification of the epidural space because the local anaesthetic subsequently injected remains undiluted, and this is important when small volumes of drug are being used. Also, a dural tap is more easily recognised if fluid has not previously been injected.

When the needle is inserted with cephalad angulation of 70°, the distance between skin and epidural space ranges between 12mm in neonates and 40mm in children of 12 years. As in the lumbar region, the "skin-to-epidural space" distance is related to age.

Paramedian approach

The technique does not greatly differ from that used in adults. The needle is inserted level with the spine immediately inferior to the space which is to be entered. The needle is directed cephalad at an angle of 45° to the long axis of the spine, and slightly medially at an angle of 5° (Fig. 69). This medial angle should be selected so that, regardless of how far laterally the needle enters the skin, the ligamentum flavum should be penetrated in the midline.

In neonates, a thick layer of fat is not infrequently found under the skin of the back. The spinous processes are therefore difficult to identify, and it is the author's opinion that, in such cases, TEA should be abandoned, since even careful probing to locate the spinous processes, as is done in adults, may be dangerous. Continuous caudal epidural with advancement of the catheter to the thoracic level may be used as an alternative in the neonate (p. 88).

Advantages

TEA allows upper abdominal surgery to be carried out without the need for muscle relaxant drugs, thus giving excellent spontaneous ventilation postoperatively and reducing the need for postoperative intensive care. The child can be returned to the ward soon after completion of

Fig. 69. The paramedian approach.

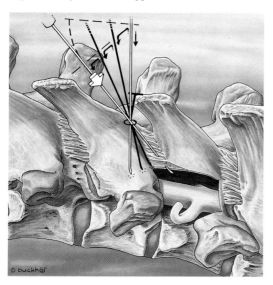

surgery and, usually, no additional analgesic or sedative drugs are required. When TEA has been used, the child is able to move his legs, in contrast to the situation after caudal and lumbar epidural anaesthesia, when motor block of the lower limbs may cause him apprehension and anxiety.

Even with blocks as high as T2, there is cardiovascular stability, with no change in the heart rate or blood pressure. As a result, vasoconstrictors are unnecessary, unless they are added to the local anaesthetic to improve motor block.

Finally, bladder dysfunction and urinary retention does not occur, and postoperative vomiting is very rare. This is probably due to the very light levels of general anaesthesia needed and to the fact that opiates can usually be avoided.

Complications

In the course of 102 cases of TEA, the author has observed no serious complications. In one neonate, the dura was punctured, but there were no sequelae. Also, in the few other published reports, no important complications were recorded. This is probably due to the fact that only anaesthetists who are fully trained and experienced in regional anaesthesia would attempt TEA in children. However, it has to be recognised that the complications reported in adults can also occur in children. In particular, direct trauma to the spinal cord and damage to the spinal arteries are possible hazards.

TEA, though useful, is a potentially dangerous technique and it should only be used in hospitals where regional anaesthesia is used routinely in children.

References

1. Schulte Steinberg O, Ostermayer R, Rahlfs VW (1984) Thoracic analgesia. Relationship between dose of etidocaine and spread of analgesia. Regional Anesthesia 9:78
2. Cousins MJ (1980) Epidural neural blockade. Edited by Cousins MJ and Bridenbaugh PO. Philadelphia. Lippincott 176

Continuous thoracic epidural block

Isabelle Murat

Continuous thoracic epidural anaesthesia should be reserved for major surgical procedures in poor risk children since in most cases it requires to be performed under general anaesthesia. Most anaesthetists working in the adult field usually perform TEA in the awake patient, but it is not reasonable to do this in children. Therefore, the block should either be performed with perfect technique by a fully trained anaesthetist highly experienced with the lumbar approach in children, or it should not be performed at all.

Furthermore the technique should be fully explained to the parents and a written informed consent should be obtained and inserted into the record of the child. The surgeon should also be informed and because of possible medico legal implications, it is important to insert a written note on the patient's record outlining the "real benefit" of the technique.

Fig. 70. Levels for thoracic epidural anaesthesia

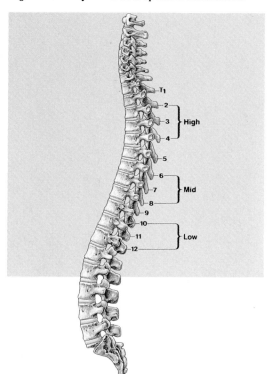

Indications

Thoracic epidural block can provide anaesthesia during the surgical procedure, and analgesia afterwards. The needle must be inserted - and the local anaesthetic deposited - at the appropriate level to produce the required band of anaesthesia (Fig 70).

1. High thoracic block involves puncture between T2 and T4, and it is required for thoracic surgery.

2. Mid-thoracic block, between T6 and T8, is required for upper abdominal surgery, because the somatic innervation of the abdomen is derived from T6 to T12.

3. Low thoracic block, between T10 and T12, is used for lower abdominal operations.

Contraindications

These are the same as for single shot thoracic epidural block.

Major abdominal surgery

In paediatric practice, continuous thoracic epidural anaesthesia is especially useful for major abdominal surgery lasting more than an hour and likely to require complete control of pain in the post-operative period. Typical examples are:

1. Nissen's fundoplication for hiatus hernia with gastro-oesophageal reflux or stenosis. The operation is often carried out on under-nourished children with respiratory disabilities (1).
2. Nephrectomy and reconstructive renal surgery.
3. Hepatectomy and surgery for biliary atresia.
4. Resection of large abdominal masses, such as Wilms tumours.

During these major surgical procedures, the sympathetic block caused by the epidural helps to reduce the stress response to surgery.

113

Post-operative period

In the post-operative period, thoracic epidural analgesia was first used in children to provide effective pain control after cardiac surgery and procedures involving sternotomy, bilateral thoracotomy and repair of coarctation of the aorta (2). It has also been used after major traumatic injuries to the thorax (3). The technique provides excellent conditions during surgery, as well as effective pain control afterwards, and this facilitates nursing procedures and physiotherapy (see chapter on post-operative analgesia).

Drugs and dosage

For children weighing less than 30kg, the recommended dose is 0.5 to 0.75ml.kg⁻¹ of 0.25% bupivacaine. This will anaesthetise a mean of 12 spinal segments, but the dose must be related to the physical condition of the child, and the level of puncture must be appropriate to the surgical procedure involved.

The mean dosages recommended here are slightly higher than those used by P. Busoni (single shot thoracic chapter). The reason for this difference is probably due to the small diameter of the catheter used. With thin catheters, it takes several minutes to inject the full dose and the distribution of solution and its longitudinal spread in the epidural space is therefore different from that when a larger needle and catheter are used.

In adults, the dose required for anaesthesia of a given number of segments by the thoracic approach is about 2/3 that required by the lumbar, because the thoracic epidural space is narrower and any injected solution therefore spreads further. This is not completely true for children, especially the very young, in whom both the anatomy of the epidural space and the nature of the epidural fat encourage the spread of local anaesthetics. In practice, therefore, the minimal dose of 0.5ml.kg⁻¹ is injected first and top-up injections are given later during surgery if necessary. In conscious adults, the extent of the block is determined by testing the number of dermatomes affected. However, in children, light general anaesthesia or benzodiazepine sedation is usually given for the operation itself, so the need for top-ups has to be determined by the child's clinical condition and the response of his monitored parameters to surgery. The volume for top-up injections is half the one which initially produced good operative conditions.

Technique

In children, continuous thoracic epidural anaesthesia is only used for major surgery. The technique itself is not always easy and can be dangerous if the patient is uncooperative. Despite this it should be done with the patient awake. General anaesthesia is to be avoided so that the patient can monitor the advancing needle by his reaction. Only in very rare, unusual situations, where a thoracic epidural block cannot be replaced by a less precarious method and where it cannot be performed on a conscious child, may general anaesthesia be considered (See also p 78).

The thoracic epidural puncture is performed with the patient in the lateral position. The prominent spine of the 7th cervical vertebra should be defined and other vertebral levels calculated from this landmark. The lower extremity of the shoulder blade is level with the 7th thoracic vertebra and this can be used as a landmark.

Both the median and paramedian approaches can be used. The median has the advantage that it is familiar to all anaesthetists. The paramedian (Fig. 71) has the advantage that the angle of entry into the epidural space can be chosen by the anaesthetist irrespective of the space available between adjacent vertebral spines, so a catheter

Fig. 71. Thoracic epidural puncture by the paramedian approach. The needle is initially directed perpendicular to the skin to ensure primary contact with the vertebral arch.

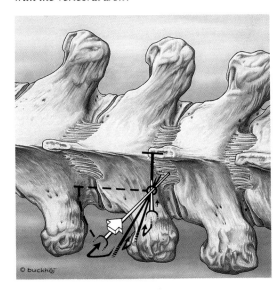

can be introduced into the epidural space in a cephalad direction without the aid of a directional bevel on the needle tip. Also, the distance of the epidural space from the skin can be easily estimated because the needle is first directed onto the vertebral lamina before being inclined cephalad to become embedded in the ligamentum flavum.

The disadvantage of the paramedian approach is that skill and experience are required if the needle is to be angled so that its tip is in the midline when it eventually enters the epidural space.

Insertion of the needle at the level of T10 to T12 is easy and the technique is the same as for the lumbar region, but the spinous processes of T10, 11 and 12 are shorter than those of the lumbar vertebrae and the spinal canal is therefore slightly more superficial (Fig 72).

The needle should be appropriate to the size and age of the child. Small Tuohy needles with a short directional bevel are available and for children of 12 kg or less, a 5cm, 19G version is suitable. For larger children, the 18G can be used. (Fig. 73). Other designs are available, including a thin-walled, 18G needle through which an 18G catheter can be passed. It has a short bevel of conventional design. The bevel is held so that it faces anteriorly. When the needle is introduced with cephalad angulation, this results in the bevel lying parallel to the epidural space and the risk of the dura being punctured by the needle tip is greatly reduced.

The thoracic epidural space can be identified by loss of resistance to normal saline or air. Air has the disadvantage that it may cause air embolism if accidental venous puncture occurs, and as it is to some extent compressible, loss of resistance is not always as definite as with saline. If saline is used, however, the injected volume should be as small as possible so that the subsequent dose of local anaesthetic is not diluted. Some workers use the 'hanging drop' method for identification of the epidural space, but this technique is more suitable for patients in the sitting position.

In children over the age of one year, the resistance offered by the ligamentum flavum is recognised without difficulty and the negative pressure of the thoracic epidural space is easily identified.

Small, 3 or 5ml syringes are suitable for young children and infants, and the 10ml size for the older patients.

When thoracic block is being performed, the needle has usually to be inserted at an acute angle to the skin due to the obliquity of the spines (Fig. 73). This is particularly noticeable when the median approach is used in the mid-thoracic

Fig. 72. Thoracic epidural puncture by the midline approach. Point of skin puncture in relation to spinous processes and angulation of needle in relation to the perpendicular plane.

Fig. 73. Entry of the needle into the thoracic epidural space. Note the position of the point in relation to the dura mater.

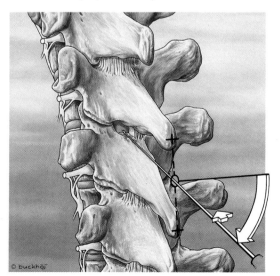

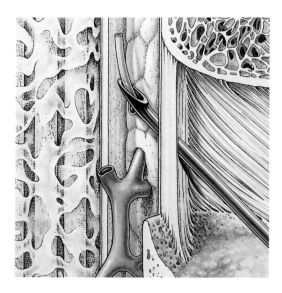

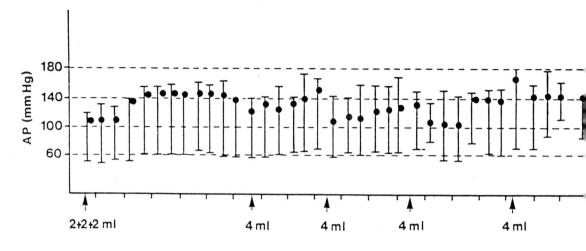

Fig 74. Thoracic epidural effect on arterial pressure.

region, but it is a feature of the paramedian approach at any level. As a result, the width of the epidural space is, in effect, increased and the position of the directional bevel is such that the needle and catheter are less likely to puncture the dura than if they had been introduced at right angles to the space by the median approach in the lumbar or lower thoracic regions. Moreover, the insertion of the catheter into the epidural space is easier and it moves cephalad freely and without resistance.

The catheter, which should be transparent, must be able to pass through the needle and this should be checked before the needle is inserted. The actual technique for insertion of the epidural catheter is the same whether the thoracic or lumbar approach is used. The catheter should pass into the thoracic epidural space without any resistance, and it should be graduated so that the exact length introduced is known. Some catheters are supplied with a stylet, which gives extra

rigidity and allows the use of thinner and less traumatic catheters. However, the stylet should only be used to assist the advance of the catheter in the needle, and it must always be withdrawn before the catheter is introduced into the epidural space.

Advance of the catheter upwards to a higher level in the epidural space is very unpredictable and cannot be guaranteed, especially in children over 6 years, as the tip of the catheter may double back on itself. 2 or 3cm are therefore usually introduced. After removal of the needle, the catheter must be securely fixed and covered with a sterile dressing such as OpSite.

An aspiration test for blood and cerebrospinal fluid should be performed before each injection. Since this does not always detect intravascular placement of the catheter, a test dose of local anaesthetic with adrenaline should be given and the effect on pulse rate and blood pressure observed.

116

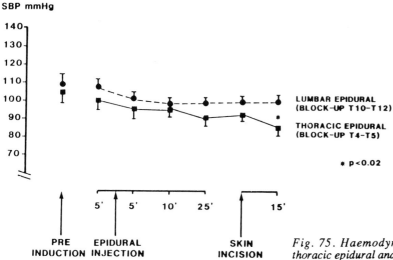

SBP mmHg

LUMBAR EPIDURAL
(BLOCK-UP T10-T12)

THORACIC EPIDURAL
(BLOCK-UP T4-T5)

* p<0.02

PRE
INDUCTION

EPIDURAL
INJECTION

SKIN
INCISION

Fig. 75. Haemodynamic effects of lumbar and thoracic epidural anaesthesia. Personal data.

Advantages

During surgery

During surgery thoracic epidural anaesthesia avoids the need for opioids and muscle relaxants, and this allows a safe and rapid recovery without the risk of respiratory depression.

It provides excellent analgesia. Although the stress response to surgery is not completely abolished, it is diminished to an extent which may be clinically significant in poorly-nourished children (8, 9).

Cardiovascular changes are minimal in children under the age of 8, even when the block extends as high as T4. Arthur (2) gave intermittent injections of bupivacaine at the T6-T7 interspace after repair of coarctation of the aorta, and could not obtain a reduction in blood pressure (Fig. 74).

Cardiovascular data from healthy children aged less than 6 receiving thoracic epidural anaesthesia were compared with a group receiving lumbar epidurals. The children were matched for age and weight, were unpremedicated and received light general anaesthesia with enflurane. They were then mechanically ventilated. In the thoracic group, the puncture level ranged between T7 and T11 and the highest level of analgesia was T4. In the lumbar group, the puncture level was L3-L4 and the highest level of anaesthesia was T10. Both groups received 0.25% bupivacaine with adrenaline 1 in 200.000 in a dose of 0.75ml.kg^{-1}

The only significant difference between them was a reduction in the systolic blood pressure 15 minutes after the skin incision in the thoracic group. This was probably due to the greater degree of sympathetic involvement and the associated reduction in compensatory vasoconstriction (Fig. 75).

Even when thoracic epidural block is combined with general anaesthesia, cardiovascular stability is such that the infusion of large volumes of intravenous fluid or the use of vasoconstrictors is not needed.

The cardiac sympathetic supply emerges from the spinal cord between C5 and T5. Epidural block extending higher than T5, therefore, has effects similar to those of B-adrenergic block, that is, decrease in cardiac rate and contractility. However, it has been shown in adults that these changes are relatively modest, and exercise tolerance is largely unaffected by high thoracic epidural block (10, 11, 12).

Blood flow to the blocked area is either maintained at its pre-block value or is increased. This is of clinical interest in visceral surgery where a good blood supply to intestinal ana-stomoses is desirable.

Post-operative period

In the post-operative period, continuous thoracic epidural analgesia can provide complete pain control where necessary (see chapter on post-operative analgesia) and this helps to prevent serious deterioration in lung function after upper abdominal and thoracic surgery (11, 12). Func-

117

tional residual capacity is more rapidly restored to normal because the patient can more easily adopt a correct posture for breathing, can inspire deeply and obtain full benefit from physiotherapy. Furthermore, high thoracic block does not itself cause adverse ventilatory changes. It has been recently shown, in adults, that resting ventilation and the ventilatory response to CO_2 are not affected by high sympathetic denervation induced by thoracic block (14, 15, 16).

A final advantage is that thoracic epidural block can decrease the duration of post-operative ileus after upper abdominal surgery (17, 18).

Complications

Since no clinically significant cardiovascular or respiratory effects occur, the most important complication of thoracic epidural anaesthesia is dural puncture, with the possibility of direct damage to the spinal cord. In view of this, the indications for the technique must be very clearly established in each case, and the block itself must only be performed by an anaesthetist experienced in the lumbar approach in children. Other complications are not specific to the thoracic route and occur with the lumbar approach also.

They include intravascular injection through needle or catheter, and haematoma and sepsis in the epidural space. No such complications have been reported in children and none has occured in the author's experience.

References

1. Meignier M, Souron R, Le Neel JC (1983) Post-operative dorsal epidural analgesia in the child with respiratory disabilities. Anesthesiology 59:473
2. Arthur DS (1980) Postoperative thoracic epidural analgesia in children. Anaesthesia 35:1131
3. Shapiro LA, Jedeikin RJ, Shalev D, Hoffman S (1984) Epidural morphine analgesia in children. Anesthesiology 61: 210
4. Tucker GT, Mather LE (1975) Pharmacokinetics of local anaesthetic agents. British Journal of Anaesthesia 47:213
5. Warner MA, Kunkel SE, Offord KO, Atchinson SR, Dawson B (1987) The effects of age, epinephrine, and operative site on duration of caudal analgesia in pediatric patients. Anesth Analg 66:995

6. Rose DK, Froese AB (1980) Changes in respiratory pattern affect dead space tidal volume ratio during spontaneous but not during controlled ventilation. A study in pediatric patients. Anesth Analg 59:341
7. Lindahl SGE, Hulse MG, Hatch DJ (1984) Ventilation and gas exchange during anaesthesia and surgery in spontaneously breathing infants and children. Brit J Anaesth 56:121
8. Håkanson E, Rutberg H, Jorfeldt L, Martensson J (1985) Effects of the extradural administration of morphine or bupivacaine on the metabolic response to upper abdominal surgery. Brit J Anaesth 57:394
9. Kehlet H (1984) The stress response to anaesthesia and surgery: release mechanisms and modifying factors. Clinics in Anaesthesiology 2:315
10. Otton PE, Wilson EJ (1966) The cardio-circulatory effects of upper thoracic epidural analgesia. Canad Anaesth' Soc J 13:541
11. Wahba WM, Craig DB, Don HF, Becklake MR (1972) The cardiorespiratory effects of thoracic epidural anaesthesia. Canad Anaesth Soc J 19:8
12. Ottesen S (1978) The influence of thoracic epidural analgesia on the circulation at rest and during physical exercise in man. Acta Anaesth Scand 22:537
13. MacCarthy GS (1976) The effect of thoracic extradural analgesia on pulmonary gas distribution, functional residual capacity and airway closure. Brit J Anaesth 48:234
14. Sjögren S, Wright B (1972) Respiratory changes during continuous epidural blockade. Acta Anaesth Scand 16:27
15. Takasaki M, Takahashi T (1980) Respiratory function during cervical and thoracic extradural analgesia in patients with normal lungs. Brit J Anaesth 52:1271
16. Dohi S, Takeshima R, Naito H (1986) Ventilatory and circulatory responses to carbon dioxide and high level sympathectomy induced by epidural blockade in awake humans. Anesth Analg 65:9
17. Aitkenhead AR, Wishart HY, Peebles Brown DA (1978) High spinal nerve block for large bowel anastomosis. Brit J Anaesth 50:177
18. Gelman S, Feigenberg Z, Dintzman M, Levy E (1977) Electroenterography after cholecystectomy. The role of high epidural analgesia. Arch Surg 112:580

Spinal block

Claude Saint-Maurice

The early application of spinal anaesthesia (3) has been outlined in the chapter on history. It continued in fairly general use in children up to the beginning of the 1960s (9-10), but the advent of the newer volatile agents, particularly halothane, and the muscle relaxants temporarily consigned the technique to oblivion. According to most authors, the principal disadvantage was that it was impossible to obtain satisfactory co-operation from the child without the use of some form of general anaesthesia, induced by an inhalational, intravenous or rectally administered agent.

Recently, some anaesthetists have shown renewed interest in this technique for use in paediatric practice (1, 4, 8, 12, 17, 19).

Before dealing with the indications, advantages and disadvantages of spinal anaesthesia in children, the technique and dosage will be considered with particular reference to the extent to which they differ from adult practice.

Fig. 76. Spinal anaesthesia.

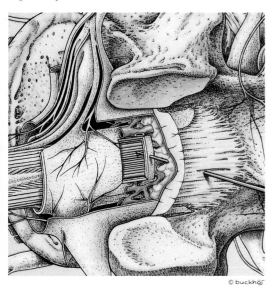

© buckhöj

Equipment

The technique differs little from that used in adults (7) except in the equipment used. The needles should be shorter (3.5 to 5 cm) than adult spinal needles, with a diameter ranging from 22 to 26G. Such needles are manufactured by several companies, including Everett in England, Vygon in France, Braun and Pajung in Germany and Sherwood and Becton Dickinson in the United States. Some anaesthetists use the internal metal needles from short percutaneous cannulae (4). The 24G Deserett cannula contains a needle of 27G diameter, and this has several advantages - the system gives perfect rigidity and easy penetration; the cerebrospinal fluid is immediately visible when it flows back because the needle hub is transparent plastic; and the length is ideally suited for use in infants (4). The lack of a stilette is a disadvantage, but this causes no difficulty if the syringe is ready for injection so that unnecessary loss of cerebrospinal fluid is eliminated.

Two types of glass syringe may be used - the 2ml size, with a Luer lock adapter, in which each interval represents 0.1ml; and the 1ml insulin syringe, which is more accurate since each interval represents 0.025ml. The latter is particularly useful for infants, in whom the volume of CSF in the needle is important and has to be allowed for when the dose is being drawn up. This volume varies from 0.01 to 0.1ml, depending on the model of needle used.

Technique

If premedication is considered necessary, it is usually given rectally (16) and incorporates a benzodiazepine in children over six months old, and atropine. Premedicated children are given general anaesthesia as described elsewhere. Newborn or infants up to 3 months do not need general anaesthesia. The child is placed in the lateral decubitus position with the side to be operated on downwards, but in the case of the newborn and infants less than three months old, the sitting position may be preferred (Fig. 77). The method of dural puncture does not differ in any way from the same procedure in an adult; in fact the flexibility of the child's spine and the ready access to the intervertebral space make it easier. The strict lateral decubitus position should be maintained and checked before the puncture is performed to ensure that the back is vertical. The needle should then be inserted exactly parallel to the table. If this is done, the principal cause of failed dural puncture is avoided.

The puncture is performed in the midline at L3-4 in children over one year and at L4-5 in infants since in this age group the spinal cord reaches down to the level of the third lumbar vertebra. An introducer is unnecessary, even for a 26G needle, because the child's skin is readily pierced, but its use does avoid the risk of skin preparation solution being carried through to the subarachnoid space.

The bevel of the needle is introduced facing laterally, parallel with the fibres, so that the fibres are separated rather than cut (Fig 79). This minimises the size of the hole.

Abajian (1) advises that in children it is better not to aspirate any cerebrospinal fluid so that the small amount of local anaesthetic is not diluted. The injection should be made slowly, in not less than 20 seconds. As a safety precaution, the syringe should contain only the exact volume of anaesthetic solution to be injected.

Fig. 77. Sitting position for infants less than three months old.

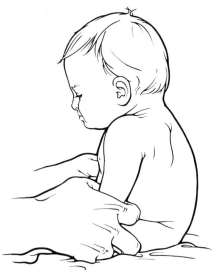

L1 1 year

L3 Newborn

S2 1 year

S4 Newborn

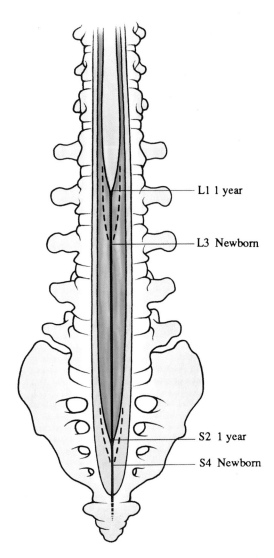

L1 1 year

L3 Newborn

S2 1 year

S4 Newborn

Fig. 78. Levels of spinal cord and spinal canal in newborn and children one year of age.

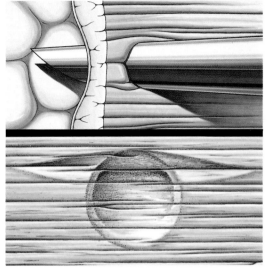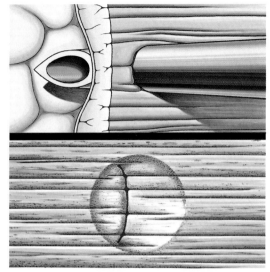

Fig. 79. The bevel of the needle introduced parallel with the fibres separates rather than cuts them.

After the needle has been withdrawn, the child is turned supine if bilateral anaesthesia is required. If a hyperbaric solution has been used, the head and thorax are raised slightly (about 15-20°), but with an isobaric solution, the child is kept absolutely flat. If unilateral anaesthesia is required, the lateral decubitus position is maintained for one minute after injection of a hyperbaric solution.

Experience has shown that this is effective in lateralising the block.

Only two minutes are required for the establishment of analgesia in infants (1). In older children the present author has found that surgery can commence after five minutes since maximum analgesia has been established within this time.

Skin-subarachnoid distance

The author has measured the depth of needle insertion at the time of local anaesthetic injection in 23 children aged from one to nine years. It is noteworthy that this depth does not correlate with age, height or weight. This finding is readily explained by the lack of precision in the measurement, in contrast to the epidural space where the end-point is very exact and the space itself only a few millimetres wide. However, the figures for the depth range from 17 to 40mm,

and this does support the view that paediatric spinal needles need not exceed 4.5-5cm. The use of a short needle allows greater accuracy of movement and ensures that the dead space is minimal - an important point in infants in whom small volumes of local anaesthetic are being injected.

Drugs and dosage

Of the several spinal agents used in adults, only tetracaine, lidocaine, bupivacaine and nupercaine have been adopted for children. Both hypobaric and hyperbaric solutions have to be considered.

Hypobaric solutions

For both the hypobaric solutions described below, the premedicated child is placed in the sitting position and a mixture of nitrous oxide (70%) and oxygen is administered. After injection, the sitting position is maintained for a period in seconds equal to the length of the spine in centimeters from the fourth lumbar vertebra to the spine of the seventh cervical vertebra. The necessity for the sitting position while the child is receiving an inhalational agent is a major disadvantage of this method (though ketamine - IV or IM - does permit the sitting position to be maintained without other equipment being required), and the complicated calculation of the period for which the child must remain sitting is somewhat unconvincing. On the other hand, the dose regime of 0.5ml of solution per year of age is rather more accurate than the hyperbaric regimes (18).

Tetracaine

Hypobaric tetracaine has been used by Slater and Stephen (18). The solution is obtained by dissolving 20mg tetracaine crystals in 20ml of double-distilled water, giving a 0.1% solution which contains 1mg per ml. The usual dose, as mentioned above, is 0.5ml (that is, 0.5mg) per year of age.

Blaise (4) suggests a 1% (10mg per ml) solution of isobaric tetracaine, but this concentration is quite unsuitable for paediatric anaes-thesia because the volumes required for infants (and even for young children) are very small and the author himself acknowledges that he cannot obtain reliable anaesthesia with volumes less than 0.2ml.

Furthermore, it is known that the subarachnoid efficiency of tetracaine is reduced when its concentration exceeds 0.5%.

Cinchocaine (Nupercaine)

Leigh (11) was the first to use hypobaric nuper-caine in a concentration of 1 in 1.500 (0.067%) for abdominal surgery in children. When the cytotoxicity of the drug is taken into account, together with the difficulties inherent in administering inhalational anaesthesia to a child in the sitting position, the use of hypobaric nupercaine cannot be recommended.

Hyperbaric solutions

Amethocaine (Tetracaine)

The mixture generally used for adults is a 1% solution obtained by dissolving 20mg tetracaine in 2ml of double-distilled water (15). For children, this solution is then diluted with an equal volume of 10% glucose to give a final concentration of 0.5% tetracaine in 5% glucose.

The dose for a T7-T10 level is 0.40 to 0.50mg.kg^{-1} for infants up to 5kg, 0.30 to 0.40 mg.kg^{-1} for children between 5 and 15kg and 0.25 to 0.30mg.kg^{-1} for children weighing more than 15kg.

Cinchocaine (Nupercaine)

Som (19) uses a 1 in 200 (0.5%, or 5mg per ml) solution in 6% glucose, but is not very precise about dose recommendations. For a child of 9kg, 0.625mg provides anaesthesia up to L1; 0.95mg to T10, and 1.25mg to T7.

For children lighter or heavier than 9kg, a proportionate dose is given, that is, double for 18kg and treble for 27kg. Hyperbaric nupercaine is now difficult if not impossible to obtain.

Tetracaine-procaine mixture

Berkowitz and Greene (5) have suggested using a slightly hyperbaric mixture obtained by preparing a 5% procaine solution, with cerebro-spinal fluid as the solvent, and diluting this with an equal volume of 1% tetracaine. This mixture therefore contains 0.5% tetracaine and 2.5% procaine and gives a more rapid onset of anal-gesia. Dosage is based on the tetracaine compo-nent of the mixture - 0.1mg per pound body weight, or 1mg per year of age.

There are obvious difficulties and risks of introducing sepsis associated with the preparation of this solution, and there are other disadvan-tages. The recommended dose regimes are im-precise because they may vary between 1 and 2 mg for a child of, say, one year; the solution is at the limit of isobaricity; and procaine is now only obtainable as a solution. Most anaesthetists therefore favour 0.5% tetracaine in 5% glucose because it is simpler and safer to prepare.

Lidocaine

Hyperbaric lidocaine can be used in children, but it is necessary to add a vasoconstrictor, such as adrenaline 1 in 200.000, in order to prolong its duration of action. Melman recommends doses of 1.5 to 2.5mg.kg^{-1}. The latter dose provides anaesthesia to T6 (13).

Bupivacaine

The present author has used hyperbaric bupiva-caine 0.5% in 8% glucose in a dose equal to that quoted above for 0.5% hyperbaric tetracaine. No statistical difference was found between the duration of action of the two agents.

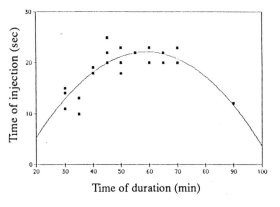

y-axis: Time of injection (sec)

x-axis: Time of duration (min)

Fig. 80. Relationship between speed of injection and duration. Saint-Maurice C, Landais A. Personal data

Addition of vasoconstrictors

As mentioned above in the case of lidocaine, vasoconstrictors are necessary to prolong the duration of spinal anaesthesia which is shorter in children than in adults. Abajian has shown that the addition of 0.01mg of adrenaline can extend the duration of analgesia by 32% in infants (1). Lower concentrations may be sufficient, as Melman recommends. The present author has found that the addition of phenylephrine at a minimal concentration of 1 in 25.000 extends the duration of analgesia from 46.4 minutes (+ or - 12.9) to 70.55 minutes (+ or - 20.53).

Doses and duration

If the recommended doses of local anaesthetic seem high, particularly for neonates and infants, it should be borne in mind that the volume of cerebrospinal fluid is proportionately twice that of the adult, being of the order of 4ml.kg^{-1} in the infant as against 2ml.kg^{-1} in adults, and that half of this volume is contained in the spinal part of the subarachnoid space. Thus the concentration of tetracaine in hyperbaric solution in the cerebrospinal fluid in a 10kg infant receiving 0.25mg.kg^{-1}, (i.e. 2.5mg,) is 0.0625mg.ml^{-1}. The equivalent in a 70kg adult would amount to 3.5mg - a very small dose. This explains why Harnik recommends average doses of 0.41mg. kg^{-1} for newborn babies weighing 2 to 3kg (8), and in fact this is occasionally insufficient.

The short duration of analgesia is very surprising. It is probably the result of more rapid absorption due to more extensive vascularisation, and not to the larger diffusion space than in the adult.

Lastly, the importance of the speed of injection in relation to duration should be noted. Rapid injection causes widespread diffusion of the solution and results in a block of short duration. The injection should extend over at least 20 seconds and for this, insulin syringes are an advantage for use in young children (Fig 80).

Level of anaesthesia

Anaesthesia is established very quickly in 2 to 4 minutes. In the conscious child, it is easily recognised by paralysis of the lower limbs. However, the actual level reached is much more difficult to define, and only tolerance of a surgical stimulus indicates that the block extends at least to the dermatomes supplying the operative area. It may be possible to pin-point the level of the block by observing signs of intercostal paralysis which become apparent when the block reaches T5. Similarly, regression of the block may be indicated by an increase in the heart rate and blood pressure, and confirmed later by movement of the lower limbs, but assessment during surgery is very imprecise.

After surgery, on the other hand, the level of block can be easily defined by testing with ice to establish the response to cold. The author has used this method and found that it is possible to predict the return of lower limb movement from the time when sensation to cold no longer affects the thoracic segments.

However, this does not make the technique applicable for day stay surgery because some difficulties, complications even, only become apparent after 24 hours, and it is therefore preferable to keep the children for at least a day.

Difficulties and accidents

Experience with spinal anaesthesia in children is still limited, and although the technique is extensively employed in adults, it is used much less in paediatric practice than caudal and epidural anaesthesia. This almost certainly explains the absence of data on accidents, since there is no obvious reason why a child should be immune to the complications observed in adults. The single exception here, all authors agree, is the cardiovascular stability which children maintain under spinal anaesthesia and other block techniques and which is due to less extensive motor paralysis.

Nevertheless, premature mobilisation should be avoided in case of syncope when the child stands up. Evidently an extension of the level of spinal anaesthesia can induce a decrease in blood pressure.

The main risk is the introduction of infection into the subarachnoid space, and this should be prevented by a strict aseptic technique. Care must be taken, however, that the skin preparation solution is not allowed to cause chemical irritation by being conveyed into the subarachnoid space on the spinal needle.

Failure to puncture the dura and obtain cerebrospinal fluid reflects the technical inexperience of the anaesthetist, as access to the subarachnoid space is usually easy. The commonest difficulty is failure to achieve an adequate block. This may be manifested as an inadequate level of analgesia, either from the outset or towards the end if surgery is delayed or continues too long. The problem can often be overcome by infiltrating with local anaesthetic, increasing the inhalational component or giving ketamine. If there is doubt as to whether the local anaesthetic will last long enough, the addition of adrenaline is an advantage.

The second most common difficulty is headache, but its incidence is hard to establish. Needle diameter is an important causal factor as it is in adults. Blaise (4) noted it in a 2 year old child after a 23g needle had been used. The present author observed two cases of headache during the course of 22 spinals in children aged 3 to 8 years, in whom 22g needles had been used.

However, when the needle size was reduced to 24, 25 and 26g, no headaches were found in 60 cases ranging from 2 to 8 years of age. Obviously, figures from such small groups can only indicate trends and cannot give an accurate incidence of this complication.

Lastly, reference should be made to two cases of apnoea, observed by Harnik and colleagues (8), involving premature babies who had exhibited the respiratory distress syndrome. One infant stopped breathing after the administration of tetracaine, though there was no evidence of extensive spread of the block. The other case, a large premature baby with a temperature of 34.2,

had an apnoea attack after 8 hours. So far as the author is aware, no other cases have been described in the literature.

In conclusion, it should be stressed that the child is not immune to the complications which occur in adults, and the standards of supervision should therefore be high.

Advantages
No other technique can provide such extensive anaesthesia with such a small volume of local anaesthetic. Spinal block is simple to perform and gives excellent muscle relaxation so it is possible to dispense with general anaesthesia in neonates and small infants. The cardiovascular system of children, at least up to the age of 8 (14), remains very stable under a spinal.

Disadvantages
Several authors (1, 2, 12) have cited the short duration of action (even when adrenaline is used) as the principal disadvantage. In this respect, the child's behaviour under spinal anaesthesia differs from the adult's, and a spinal cannot be expected to provide prolonged post-operative analgesia. The risk of headache should not be exaggerated since the incidence can be reduced considerably by sound technique and the use of small-diameter needles.

Indications
Spinal block certainly has a place in paediatric regional anaesthesia. It can be used with advantage for operations of short duration (up to 45 minutes, or 60 minutes if a vasoconstrictor is used) in the sub-umbilical region. It is therefore suitable for abdominal procedures such as appendicectomy and inguinal herniotomy, and for surgery of the external genitalia and lower limb. The age groups most likely to benefit are neonates and young premature infants who have suffered from the respiratory distress syndrome and who are known to be at risk of apnoea attacks after general anaesthesia. The complete lower limb paralysis produced by a spinal greatly facilitates the operating table management of these infants to whom no general anaesthetic is administered.

Lastly, spinal anaesthesia is safe and cheap, and it therefore has a possible part to play, together with other regional techniques, in countries where standards of anaesthetic equipment are still far below those enjoyed by the developed countries.

Contraindications

These fall into two categories: the general contra-indications, mentioned elsewhere in this book, concerned with septicaemia, bacteraemia and coagulopathies; and the local contraindications, such as infections at the site of needle puncture and affecting skin, muscle or vertebrae.

References

1. Abajian JC, Mellish PWI, Browne AE, Perkins FM, Lambert DH, Mazuzian JE (1984) Spinal anesthesia for the high risk infant. Anesth Analg 63:359
2. Armitage EN (1985) Regional anaesthesia in Paediatrics. Clinics in Anaesthesiology 3: 553
3. Bainbridge WS (1901) Report 712. Operations on infants and young children under spinal anaesthesia. Arch Pediatr 18: 510
4. Blaise G (1984) Spinal anesthesia in children. Anesth Analg 63:1139
5. Berkowitz S, Greene BA (1951) Spinal anesthesia in children. Report based on 350 patients under 13 years of age. Anesthesiology 12, 3: 376
6. Calvert DG (1966) Direct spinal anesthesia for repair of myelomeningocoele. B J A 2, 5505:86
7. Etherington-Wilson (1945) Spinal anaesthesia in the very young and further observations. Pr Roy Soc Med 38:109
8. Harnik EV, Hoy GR, Potolicchio S, Steward DJ, Siegelman RE (1986) Spinal anesthesia in premature infants recovering from respiratory distress syndrome. Anesthesiology 64:95
9. Junkin CI (1933) Spinal anesthesia in children. Canad Med Am J 28:51
10. Leigh MD, Belton MK (1960) Pediatr Anesth New York - The MacMillan Co
11. Leigh MD (1943) Spinal anesthesia in infants and children. Int Anesthesiology Clinics 1-3, Boston, Little, Brown and Co.
12. Mathew JI, Moreno L (1984) Spinal anesthesia for high risk neonates. Anesth Analg 63:782
13. Melman E, Penuelas J, Marrufo J (1975) Regional anesthesia in children. Current Researches 54:387
14. Murat I, Delleur MM, Esteve C, Egu JF, Raynaud P, Saint-Maurice CI. (1987) Continuous epidural anaesthesia in children: clinical and haemodynamic implications. Br J Anaesth 59:1441
15. Saint-Maurice CI. Rachianesthesie. Encycl Med Chir Paris, Anesthésie-Réanimation, 4-2-09, Fasc 36324 A10: 1
16. Saint-Maurice CI, Egu JF, Lepaul M, Berg a et JP Loose (1985) La préparation de l'enfant à l'anesthésie générale - JEPU Anesthésie-Réanimation - Arnette, Paris
17. Schulte Steinberg O (1988) Neural blockade for pediatric surgery in Neural blockade in Clinical Anesthesia and Pain Management. MJ Cousins and PO Bridenbaugh Lippincott - Philadelphia
18. Slater HM, Stephen CR (1950) Hypobaric pontocaine spinal anesthesia in children. Anesthesiology 11, 6:709
19. Som MM (1984) Spinal anesthesia in Pediatrics Indian J Anaesth 12, 1:86
20. Weisman LE, Merenstein GB, Steenbarger Jr (1983) The effect of lumbar puncture position in sick neonates. Am J Dis Child 137:107

Peripheral nerve blocks

Ottheinz Schulte Steinberg

Introduction

The anatomy and general principles of peripheral nerve blocks are the same in children and adults. A clear understanding of the regional anatomy is essential, with particular reference to fascial, aponeurotic and muscle layers. These can be easily identified with a short-bevelled needle and they help the anaesthetist to assess depth and to deposit local anaesthetic around the nerve in the correct tissue plane. As depth is the parameter which varies most with age, these anatomical depth markers are invaluable when blocks are being performed in children. When a child is under general anaesthesia and cannot indicate when the needle is near to a nerve, an electrical nerve stimulator is also an invaluable aid. The newer instruments operate at low current levels with pulses of ultrashort duration and only cause motor stimulation without paraesthesia when the needle tip is very close to the nerve. They may prove to be of help in preventing nerve injury by needle trauma.

The nerves of neonates and infants are incompletely myelinated and those of children are relatively thin. Local anaesthetic drugs therefore penetrate even the larger nerves rapidly, and small doses of comparatively dilute solutions produce adequate blocks.

For prolonged procedures and for postoperative analgesia, long-acting local anaesthetic agents are required, whereas for outpatients, an agent of shorter duration might be preferred. Blocks of the larger nerves, such as the sciatic and the brachial plexus, require larger volumes of solution (the same volume for both procedures), but close attention has then to be paid to the maximum dose, particularly when these blocks are combined with other regional techniques. Adequate volumes are essential to reach the nerves. It can be achieved by diluting the solution when maximum doses have been reached.

The local anaesthetic solutions used are 2% 2-chloroprocaine, 0,7-1% lidocaine or mepivacaine and bupivacaine 0,19-0,25%. The concentration of 0,19% is obtained by adding one part of water or saline to three parts of 0,25% bupivacaine.

126

Blocks of the upper limb

Ottheinz Schulte Steinberg

General remarks

Light general anaesthesia, preceded by normal premedication, is more likely to be necessary for the block to be performed in children, and the plexus is then located with an electrical nerve stimulator. However, in some cases, such as after a fracture, the conscious child may well tolerate a pain- relieving block. Upper limb blocks may also be performed in the awake child if he is cooperative and old enough, and in these cases, a light benzodiazepine premedication is given. The child can assist in monitoring paraesthesiae although with modern nerve stimulators these are not required.

Fig. 81. Four approaches to the brachial plexus.

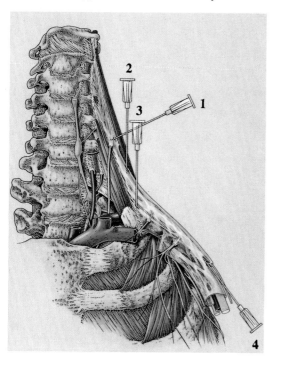

Anatomy

The brachial plexus is derived from the ventral rami of C5 to T1. C4 and T2 also send small branches to the plexus. The roots enter an ensheathed space between scalenus anterior and scalenus medius, the so-called interscalene space. The sheath enveloping the plexus extends from the transverse processes of the cervical vertebrae down as far as the axilla. As they run distally, the roots converge to form three trunks (upper, middle and lower) and they are accompanied anteriorly and medially by the subclavian artery. Behind the clavicle, the trunks divide into anterior and posterior divisions which pass over the first rib, together with the artery, and, at the level of the second part of the axillary artery, form cords by uniting again. The cords give rise to the nerves which supply the outer surface of the upper arm, the shoulder joint, the forearm and the hand. The inside of the upper arm is supplied from T2 which is not normally contained in the brachial plexus. The cutaneous innervation of the shoulder and supraclavicular area is supplied by the cervical plexus (C3-4).

The brachial plexus can be approached by four routes (Fig. 81):

1. Interscalene, described by Winnie (1) and Miranda (2)
2. Subclavian perivascular, described by Winnie (1)
3. Supraclavicular, described by Fortin (3)
   These approaches are at the level of roots and trunks.

4. Axillary

Here, the nerves of the plexus leave the neuromuscular sheath which has accompanied them distally, and they now become grouped round the axillary artery, with the median and musculocutaneous nerves above it, the ulnar medial to it and the radial behind. It is important to note that the musculocutaneous nerve leaves the axillary sheath at the level of the coracoid process and may escape block by the axillary route.

127

Indications

Of the techniques mentioned above, the axillary is the most popular for children. However, the site of block should be determined with due regard for the site of operation. For operations on the forearm and the outer aspect of the upper arm, including reduction of a dislocated shoulder, the anaesthetist should choose one of the first three techniques. With the additional block of the superficial cervical plexus and subcutaneous infiltration of the areas supplied by the inter-costobrachial and medial brachial cutaneous nerves, it is even possible to provide adequate anaesthesia for open shoulder surgery.

The axillary approach is indicated for operations on the medial side of the forearm and hand. However, it has the highest failure rate because the musculocutaneous nerve, which supplies the radial aspect of the forearm and the base of the thumb, is not always blocked.

Contraindications

The usual contraindications to regional blocks apply. Contralateral paresis of the phrenic and recurrent laryngeal nerves are contraindications to the interscalene and supraclavicular approaches because, if the ipsilateral nerves are anaes-thetised, bilateral paresis will result. Haemorr-hage is a risk during the supraclavicular approach due to the proximity of the subclavian artery, so it is particularly important to exclude any haemorrhagic diathesis. Similarly, pneumo-thorax is also a risk and a pre-existing contra-lateral pneumothorax is a contraindication.

The axillary approach is contraindicated when the arm cannot be abducted to 90° because it may then be impossible to palpate the landmarks or to insert the needle correctly. The presence of infected axillary glands is also a contraindication.

Equipment

One or two 20ml syringes, an extension set (Fig. 82), a short-bevel 23g needle, a 25g needle for local infiltration and a nerve stimulator with attachments should be available, but not all these items will be required for every block.

Fig. 82. "Immobile needle", this system prevents movements of the needle (1).

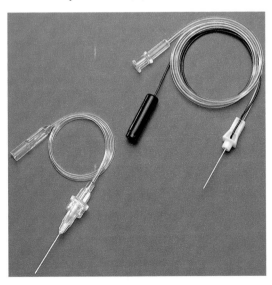

128

Drugs and dosage

The choice of drug is to some extent determined by the expected duration of the surgical procedure. For operations lasting less than one hour, 2% 2-chloroprocaine may be used. Lido-caine or mepivacaine are suitable for surgery lasting 1 1/2 to 2 hours, and for procedures lasting longer than three hours, bupivacaine is indicated.

Since four major nerves are involved in brachial plexus block regardless of where the injection is made, it is possible to devise a simplified dose regime which is applicable to all the techniques. This regime can also be used for calculating the dose for a sciatic nerve block.

Adrenaline added to local anaesthetic solutions has the effect of prolonging the duration of action, and decreasing the rate of absorption into the systemic circulation. It also decreases the onset time and intensifies motor block. If these effects are desired, adrenaline-containing solutions should be used.

Complications

Any injection administered through an infected area is likely to spread the infection to deeper tissues, and an injection given without due regard for aseptic skin preparation may also introduce infection. Also, an injection is a "blind" technique and occasional vascular damage, causing haematoma formation, is inevitable. Therefore, blocks should not be performed on patients who are known to have coagulation disorders.

Another important complication concerns absolute and relative overdosage. No technique is safe if too much drug is administered or if the correct amount of drug is injected into the wrong place. Failure to appreciate this will lead to symptoms and signs of local anaesthetic toxicity, and this is of particular importance for interscalene and supraclavicular blocks where accidental injection of even a small dose of local anaesthetic into the vertebral artery may produce catastrophic cerebral effects.

Total spinal or high (cervical) epidural anaesthesia may also occur as a complication of interscalene block, and pneumothorax may be produced with either supraclavicular or perivascular subclavian blocks.

Almost all the blocks described for the upper limb involve eliciting paraesthesiae, as these indicate when the needle is close to a nerve.

Needle trauma to the nerve is therefore a possibility with these techniques. The use of a nerve stimulator provides useful information about the position of the needle tip, and so helps to reduce damage, but it must not be relied upon to eliminate it entirely.

Side effects

Block of the stellate ganglion, recurrent laryngeal and phrenic nerves are recognised side effects of the interscalene and supraclavicular approaches, but they can be avoided if the needle is directed sufficiently caudad. They are not usually of great clinical importance.

Table 11. Simplified dose regime for brachial plexus blocks. From E. Lanz, Blockaden des Plexus brachialis im Kindesalter, in: Regionalanaesthesie im Kindes-alter, ed. K. Kuhn and J. Hausdorfer. Springer Verlag, Berlin, Heidelberg, New York, Tokyo 1984 (4).

B=Bupivacaine, L=Lidocaine, M=Mepivacaine

| Age (yrs) | Volume (ml) | | Concentration (%) | |
			L and M	B
0-4	Height (cm)	/12	0.7 - 0.8	0.19
5-8	Height (cm)	/10	0.8 - 0.9	0.25
9-16	Height (cm)	/7	0.9 - 1	0.25

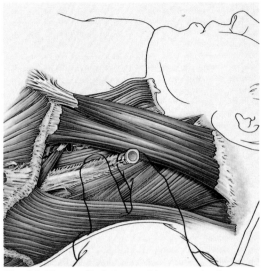

Fig. 83. *The needle is inserted between the fingers which mark the interscalene groove.*

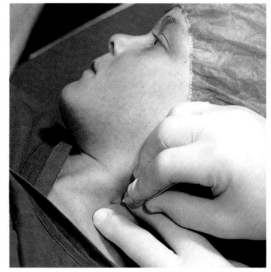

Fig. 84. *Clinical application of Fig. 83.*

Interscalene approach

Technique

The patient lies on his back with his head extended and turned slightly away from the side to be blocked. The interscalene space is located at the level of the cricoid cartilage (C6), the transverse process of which can be easily palpated only a few millimetres from the surface. Its depth from the skin gives important information to the anaesthetist.

In the conscious child, a skin wheal of local anaesthetic is raised at this point with the 25G needle attached to the extension set. This should be done slowly to minimise pain. The 23G needle is then attached and inserted through the skin wheal in a direction which is mainly medial, but also 45° caudad and slightly backward (posterior). It is most important to remember that the transverse process is very superficial and that puncture of the dura or of the vertebral artery is easy if the needle is inserted too deep.

Paraesthesiae should be elicited in the superficial part of the interscalene space and, if the needle is correctly positioned, they should be felt in the thumb, or if a nerve stimulator is being used, the contractions should be seen in the wrist or fingers.

Following a negative aspiration test, a small test dose of local anaesthetic is injected to exclude a total spinal or an accidental vertebral artery injection which would cause central nervous system signs.

If analgesia of the shoulder region is required, upward extension of the block into the cervical plexus can be facilitated by compression of the interscalene space below the tip of the needle. The interscalene approach produces no anaesthesia of the ulnar nerve in about 50% of cases. A separate ulnar nerve block may be required if analgesia in this area is needed.

Miranda technique

Miranda (2) has described a technique which does not depend on paraesthesiae. The needle is inserted into the interscalene groove at the level of the cricoid cartilage and is advanced downwards at an angle of 45° until loss of resistance is felt. This indicates that the needle has penetrated the fibrous sheath which encloses the interscalene space. It is important to use a short-bevel needle so the loss of resistance is easier to feel. The correct position of the needle now has to be confirmed. One or two ml of local anaesthetic are injected and the syringe is immediately disconnected from the needle. Some back flow will be observed if the needle is in the interscalene space since there is transient positive pressure as the potential space is opened up. No back flow is seen if the injection is made into tissues. Although paraesthesiae are not required, they can be produced by the injection of ice-cold saline. Once the correct position of the needle has been confirmed, the full anaesthetic dose can be injected.

Conclusion

Interscalene block can be performed even in obese children and abduction of the arm is not necessary. Miranda´s variation is well suited for children as it does not depend on paraesthesiae.

Fig. 85. Supraclavicular technique. The needle is inserted at the midpoint of the clavicle.

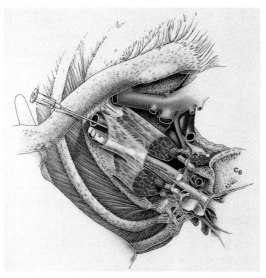

Supraclavicular approach
Technique

Fortin (3) has described the following method in which contact with the first rib - an essential part of the traditional Kulenkampff technique - is not required, so the incidence of pneumothorax is reduced. The rib in fact acts only as a protective shield for the dome of the lung.

Proper positioning of the patient is a prerequisite for success. A rolled towel is placed longitudinally between the shoulders and along the spine of the supine patient, and the shoulders are pushed backwards on to the mattress and down (caudad) towards the feet. This has the effect of moving the first rib forward towards the skin and bringing the brachial plexus and subclavian artery closer to the surface. Both the rib and the artery are easily palpable in children. The head of the patient is turned to the contralateral side.

The 25G, 1.3cm needle is attached to the extension tube and a skin wheal is raised (slowly, and therefore less painfully) 1cm above the midpoint of the clavicle just lateral to, and behind, the artery (Fig. 85). The needle is exchanged for a similar, but blunt, one and then inserted through the skin wheal and advanced slowly caudad, slightly medial and also backward. Paraesthesiae are sought by probing strictly in an anteroposterior direction without any medial or lateral deviation. Paraesthesiae or muscle contractions - when a nerve stimulator is used - are obtained very superficially. Contact with the first rib confirms the injection site, but indicates that the needle has been inserted too deeply. When the first paraesthesia has been elicited, the total dose of local anaesthetic is injected.

Subclavian perivascular approach

Technique

The patient is placed in the supine position, similar to the Fortin supraclavicular approach, except that the rolled towel is not necessary. The head is turned to the contralateral side and the subclavian artery - easily palpable in children - is located. The first rib is also easy to feel and may facilitate orientation.

The 25G needle is attached to the extension set. The palpating index finger identifies the interscalene groove at the level of the cricoid (C6) and slides down in the groove until the pulse of the subclavian artery is felt (Fig. 86). The skin wheal is raised slowly just above the palpating finger within the interscalene groove. The 23G needle is now attached and advanced in a caudad direction with the hub in line with the ear and the shaft parallel with the course of the scalenus muscles (Fig. 87). This approach results in the needle entering the interscalene space, with a 'click', at the level of C7. Paraesthesiae should be found superficially, just dorsolateral to the artery. If an aspiration test is negative, the total dose of local anaesthetic may be given provided that the paraesthesia was felt in the region to be operated on. Otherwise, an increment is injected and the rest is given as further paraesthesiae are found. When a nerve stimulator is used, the total dose is injected when appropriate muscle contractions are obtained.

The Kulenkampff technique should not be used in children because it involves deliberate probing of the first rib. With the proximity of the lung and the short distances between structures in children, the risks of producing a pneumothorax must be greater compared with other supraclavicular methods.

Conclusion

The blocks described above are the most effective methods for producing anaesthesia of the upper extremity (5).

Fig. 86. The palpating finger is moved down the interscalene groove and should feel the pulsation of the subclavian artery at this point.

Fig. 87. The needle is inserted above the palpating finger.

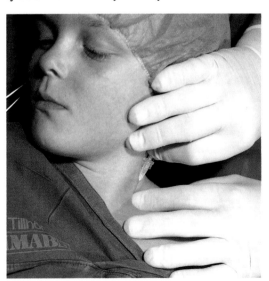

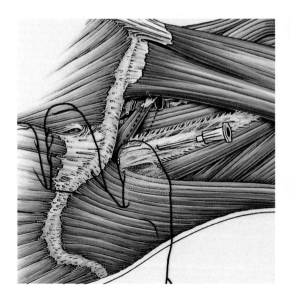

Axillary approach

Technique

The technique is essentially the same as for adults. The child is placed in the supine position with the arm abducted and externally rotated. The right handed anaesthetist palpates the axillary artery with the fingers of his left hand and presses it against the humerus at the point of conjunction of the pectoralis major and the coracobrachialis muscles (Figs. 88 and 89). With his right hand, he inserts the 25G needle attached to an extension set and slowly raises a skin wheal over the pulsating artery. The 23G needle is then attached, inserted through the skin wheal and angled cephalad towards the artery. It is advanced slowly until the needle starts to pulsate or until paraesthesiae are obtained. The muscle contractions resulting from the paraesthesiae may be recognised by an assistant holding the hand or arm of the child.

Paraesthesiae can also be provoked by the injection of ice-cold saline or by the use of a nerve stimulator. Local anaesthetic is injected from a 20ml syringe, when the position of the needle has been confirmed and after a negative aspiration test.

Fig. 88. Clinical application of Fig. 89.

After the injection, the axillary sheath distal to the injection site is kept compressed for 3 to 5 minutes and the arm is adducted. This prevents the solution from running peripherally and helps to promote its proximal spread so that the block hopefully includes the musculocutaneous nerve. If a tourniquet is to be used, a skin wheal should be raised on withdrawal of the needle to block the intercosto-brachial and medial brachial cutaneous nerves.

A catheter can be inserted into the axillary sheath for the provision of continuous anaesthesia.

Block failures

Complete or partial failure of brachial plexus blocks does occur. If there is no time to correct the situation, a general anaesthetic may have to be added. If more time is available, the extent of analgesia should be determined and, if indicated, the block may be repeated. If there are specific unblocked areas, the nerves supplying these areas can be blocked more peripherally, and some short notes on these supplementary blocks are given below.

Fig. 89. With the index finger on the pulse of the axillary artery at the junction of pectoralis major and coracobrachialis muscles a 25G needle is inserted just superior to the palpating finger tip.

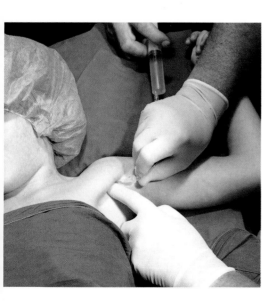

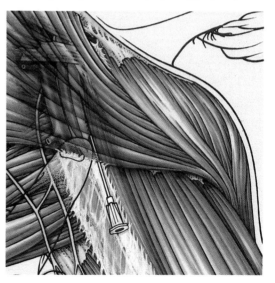

Ulnar nerve block

Anatomy

The ulnar nerve often remains unaffected after interscalene block and a supplementary block is required. The best site for this is at the elbow, where the nerve is found in the groove between the medial epicondyle of the humerus and the olecranon process of the ulna (Fig. 90).

Technique

The patient lies in the supine position with the arm across his trunk, internally rotated and flexed at the elbow. After suitable skin preparation, a skin wheal is raised midway between the tip of the olecranon and the medial epicondyle. A 23G blunt needle is then introduced in a caudad direction, almost parallel with the nerve, until a paraesthesia is obtained. (Fig. 91) 1-5ml of local anaes-thetic is injected, depending on the age of the child.

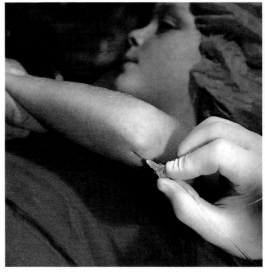

Fig. 91. Clinical application to Fig. 90.

Fig. 90. Injection of the ulnar nerve at the elbow.

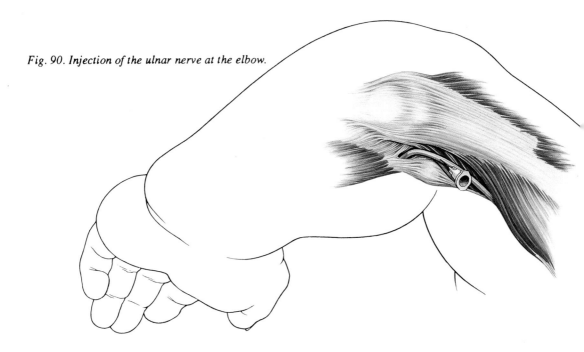

Median nerve block

Anatomy
At the elbow, this nerve lies just medial to the brachial artery (Fig. 92).

Technique
The patient lies supine with the elbow extended and the arm slightly abducted. A line is drawn between the the lateral and medial epicondyles of the humerus. After skin preparation, a skin wheal is raised on this line, immediately medial to the brachial artery. A 23G blunt needle is then inserted and paraesthesiae should be obtained at a superficial level. 1-5ml of local anaesthetic is injected, depending on the age of the child.

Radial nerve block

Anatomy
The nerve passes between the brachialis and the brachioradialis muscles anterior to the lateral condyle, and it is blocked at this site.

Technique (6)
The patient lies in the supine position with the elbow extended and the arm slightly abducted. The intercondylar line is marked and a skin wheal is raised 1-2cm lateral to the point where the biceps tendon crosses this line. A 23G blunt needle is inserted through the wheal and advanced all the way to the lateral aspect of the lateral condyle. 2-4ml of local anaesthetic are injected as the needle is slowly withdrawn almost to the skin. This manoeuvre is repeated twice, with the needle being inserted slightly less laterally each time.

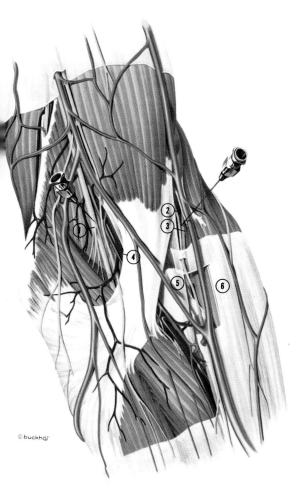

© buckhöj

Fig. 92. Anatomical landmarks for median and radial nerve blocks at the elbow.

1. Median nerve
2. Lateral cutaneous nerve of the forearm
3. Radial nerve
4. Brachial artery
5. Tendon of biceps muscle
6. Brachioradialis muscle

135

Wrist block

Nerve blocks at the wrist may be useful in children for supplementation of inadequate brachial plexus block (Fig. 93), but will probably be used rarely. A circular line around the wrist at the level of the ulnar styloid is helpful for the block.

Median nerve

Anatomy
The median nerve lies behind and slightly to the radial side of the palmaris longus tendon and medial to the tendon of the flexor carpi radialis.

Technique
The median nerve is blocked by inserting the needle vertically on the drawn line, close to the lateral border of the palmaris longus. If this tendon is absent a point medial to the ulnar edge of the flexor carpi radialis tendon on the circular line is chosen. The needle has to pierce the deep fascia and in the awake child a paraesthesia should be obtained or muscle contractions observed when a nerve stimulator is used.

1-2 ml of local anaesthetic solution is sufficient for this block.

Ulnar nerve

Anatomy
The ulnar nerve lies under cover of, and just lateral to, the flexor carpi ulnaris tendon, and on the ulnar side of, and deep to, the ulnar artery. At this point it has already given off the palmar cutaneous and dorsal branches (Fig. 94).

Technique
The block of the deep portion is performed by inserting the needle on the drawn line on the ulnar side of the flexor carpi ulnaris tendon passing through and under it. Paraesthesias may be obtained or muscle contractions observed when a nerve stimulator is used. The dorsal cutaneous branch is blocked by redirecting the needle superficially for subcutaneous infiltration along the drawn line to the middle of the back of the wrist.

Fig. 94.
1. Median nerve
2. Tendon of the flexor carpi radialis muscle
3. Tendon of palmaris longus muscle
4. Ulnar artery
5. Ulnar nerve
6. Tendon of the flexor carpi ulnaris muscle

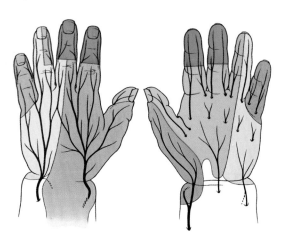

Fig. 93. The innervation of the hand.

Ulnar nerve
Median nerve
Radial nerve

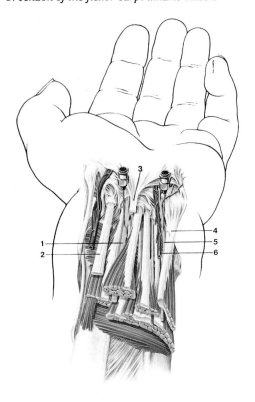

Radial nerve

Anatomy
The radial nerve lies in the subcutaneous tissue and divides just above the wrist into two branches, which supply the skin of the radial side of the dorsum of the hand and proximal parts of the radial three and one half fingers.

Technique
The radial nerve is blocked by a subcutaneous semi-circular infiltration on the previously drawn circular line starting at the lateral side of the wrist, just lateral to the radial artery. This infiltration is carried around to the back of the radial half of the wrist (Fig 95). It requires 4-6 ml of local anaesthetic solution in the small child and 10-15 ml in the older age group.

Digital nerve block

Anatomy
Terminal branches of the radial and ulnar nerves supply the back of the fingers as dorsal nerves. The palmar surface of the fingers is supplied by volar nerves consisting of terminal elements of the median and ulnar nerves.

Technique
Skin wheals are raised at the interdigital folds and a ring of local anaesthetic is then deposited around the base of the finger (Fig 96). This results in anaesthesia distal to the ring. It is important that the local anaesthetic solution does **not** contain adrenaline because this may cause gangrene. 0.5-1.5 ml of local anaesthetic, depending on the age of the child, should not be exceeded.

Fig. 96. Digital nerve block.

1. Dorsal digital nerve
2. Palmar digital nerve

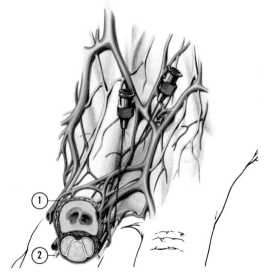

Fig. 95. Radial nerve block.

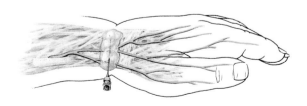

References

1. Winnie A.P.(1970) Interscalene brachial plexus block. Anesth. Analg, (Cleve) 49:455

2. Miranda D.R.(1977), Continuous brachial plexus block. Acta Anaesth Belg 4:323.

3. Fortin G. and Tremblay L.(1959), The short needle technique in brachial plexus block. Canad. Anaesth. Soc. J. 6:32.

4. Lanz E.(1984), Blockaden des Plexus brachialis im Kindesalter, in: Regionalanaesthesie im Kindesalter, ed. Kuhn, K. and Hausdorfer, J. Springer Verlag Berlin, Heidelberg, New York, Tokyo.

5. Moore D.C (1984), Regional Block, p237, Ill. Charles C. Thomas. Publisher, Springfield,

6. Berry F.R. and Bridenbaugh L.D.: The upper extremity: Somatic blockade in: Neural Blockade, p310,J.B. Lippincott Co, Philadelphia, Toronto.

7. Principles and Practice of Regional Anaesthesia (1987), ed. Wildsmith J.A.W. and Armitage E.N. Churchill Livingstone, Edinburgh, London, Melbourne and New York.

8. Techniques of Regional Anaesthesia (1989), D Bruce Scott, Mediglobe. Fribourg.

Blocks of the lower limb

T C Kester Brown

Introduction

Nerve blocks of the lower limb may be useful in paediatric practice. They may be adequate on their own, but a local block combined with caudal anaesthesia is an alternative which should be considered if regional anaesthesia is desirable.

Key anatomical points relating to the performance of the blocks will be discussed, but as the blocks are essentially similar to those used in adults, major textbooks on the subject should be consulted for more details (1, 2, 3, 4, 5). The main difference in children is that the nerves are not situated so deeply. The feeling of loss of resistance as fascia is penetrated helps to identify depth for many of the blocks discussed. A nerve stimulator may also be helpful in confirming the location of some nerves, particularly the sciatic, tibial and common peroneal.

Contraindications

There are no contraindications specific to the blocks to be described.

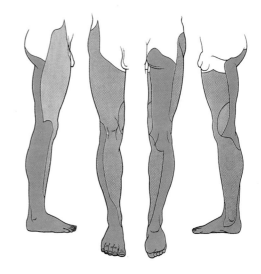

Fig. 97. Innervation of the lower limb

Sciatic nerve

Femoral nerve

Obturator nerve

Lateral cutaneous nerve

Femoral nerve block and 3 in 1 block

Anatomy

The femoral nerve, derived from the roots of L2, 3 & 4, supplies the skin on the front of the thigh and medial aspect of the leg (Fig 99). It is formed from the lumbar plexus and descends under the fascia iliaca into the femoral canal where it is encased in a sheath continuous with this fascia. Below the inguinal ligament, fascia lata covers the thigh. It also covers the femoral nerve and the femoral vessels, which lie immediately medial to the nerve.

Indications

It is a useful block for the acute management of fractured shaft of femur because it relieves pain and muscle spasm in the thigh. Because it is easy to perform in conscious children, this block can provide analgesia during X-ray examination. It also allows manipulation and immobilisation of the fracture and should be used more widely for this purpose. Femoral nerve block can also be used when donor skin is taken from the front of the thigh.

Drugs

Bupivacaine is used in a concentration of 0.3 - 0.5% and is given in a dose of about $0.3ml.kg^{-1}$ (6). A larger volume of the dilute solution is given if a 3 in 1 block is required.

Technique

A short-bevel or blunt needle is inserted immediately lateral to the femoral artery. Loss of resistance is felt twice - once when the needle penetrates the fascia lata and again when it penetrates the fascia iliaca. It should now lie in the canal containing the femoral nerve. The vessels, in contrast, lie superficial to the fascia iliaca.

If a 3 in 1 block is being performed, the femoral canal is compressed distal to the injection site (7). This encourages the local anaesthetic to spread upwards under the fascia iliaca so that the lateral cutaneous and obturator nerves are blocked as well as the femoral.

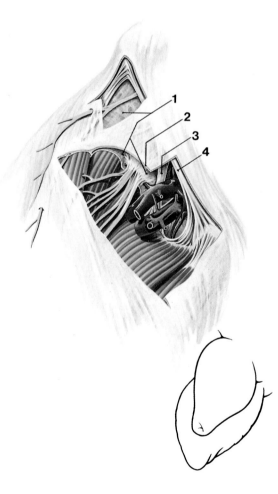

Fig. 98.

1. Fascia iliaca
2. Fascia lata
3. Fascia interlagunare
4. Inguinal ligament

Block of lateral cutaneous nerve of the thigh

Anatomy
The lateral cutaneous nerve of the thigh (L2-3) passes down under the fascia iliaca to emerge under the inguinal ligament just medial and inferior to the anterior superior iliac spine, deep to the fascia lata. Immediately medial to the anterior superior iliac spine, it lies in a canal deep to the external oblique aponeurosis and the insertion of the internal oblique muscle.

Indications
Block of this nerve can provide analgesia for incisions on the lateral aspect of the thigh or when donor skin is taken in that region. It is also a useful block during hip surgery for which a coloured dye is added to the local anaesthetic and for which an approach immediately medial to the anterior superior iliac spine is used. As well as providing analgesia, this outlines the route of the nerve below the inguinal ligament and assists the surgeon in preserving it.

Drugs
Bupivacaine 0.25% in a dose of 2 - 5ml.

Techniques
1. If a needle is inserted immediately medial to the anterior superior iliac spine, loss of resistance can be felt as the needle penetrates the external oblique aponeurosis and again when it emerges from the internal oblique muscle and enters the canal carrying the nerve. There is resistance to injection while the needle is passing through the muscle (8).
2. An alternative approach is to insert the needle about 2cm below and just medial to the anterior superior iliac spine. Loss of resistance is felt as the fascia lata is penetrated and local anaesthetic injected here will usually bathe the nerve.
3. A third approach is to insert the needle as in 2, but to direct it up under the inguinal ligament just medial to the anterior superior iliac spine.

Block of posterior cutaneous nerve of the thigh

Anatomy
The nerve is derived from the first, second and third sacral roots and it supplies the lower part of the buttock, the perineum and the back of the thigh. It diverges from the sciatic nerve deep to the gluteus maximus muscle and emerges to become cutaneous below its lower medial border.

Indications
Block of this nerve is mainly used when donor skin is taken from the back of the thigh.

Drugs
5 - 15ml of 0.25% bupivacaine are used for this block.

Technique
The posterior cutaneous nerve of the thigh can be blocked with the posterior approach to the sciatic nerve or as a separate procedure in which the branches of the nerve are blocked as they emerge from the lower border of the gluteus maximus.

The landmark for this block is the gluteal fold just below a point one quarter of the distance from the ischial tuberosity to the greater trochanter. The patient lies prone, or supine with the leg raised, and resistance is felt as the needle is passed through the superficial fascia and then through a deeper fibrous fatty layer. Loss of resistance will be felt as the needle emerges from both these layers and injection becomes easy as the needle enters the space in which the nerves lie. Depending on the size of the child, 5-15ml of local anaesthetic should be injected because several ramifying branches must be anaesthetised, unlike a single nerve in a confined space (9).

Obturator nerve block

As is the case in adults, this nerve is rarely blocked on its own in children, but it is included with the femoral and the lateral cutaneous nerve of the thigh in the 3 in 1 block.

Indications

The obturator nerve supplies mainly the adductor muscles of the hip and a block can serve as a diagnostic test to see whether benefit might be obtained from surgical intervention in certain spastic conditions.

Technique

The needle is inserted lateral to and below the pubic tubercle and is advanced until it contacts the inferior pubic edge.

1. The depth is noted and the needle is withdrawn and directed cephalad 45° and advanced until it hits the superior pubic edge.

2. The needle is withdrawn and reinserted at an angle half way between these to a depth deeper than the previous insertion (2 cm in adults).

3. The tip of the needle should now be in the obturator canal. The distances have to be reduced proportionally in children and a dose of 1 to 5 ml of local anaesthetic is injected after an aspiration test as there are vessels in the area.

Fig. 99. Obturator nerve block.

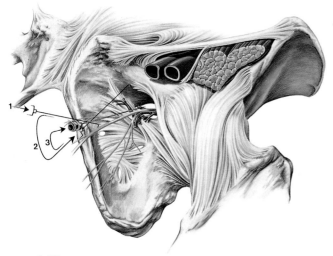

Fig. 100. Obturator nerve L2-4

1. *Anterior branch*
2. *Posterior branch*
3. *Pectineus muscle*
4. *Adductor brevis muscle*
5. *Adductor longus muscle*
6. *Gracilis muscle*
7. *Cutaneous branch*
8. *Branch to the hip joint*
9. *Adductor magnus muscle*
10. *Branch to the knee joint*

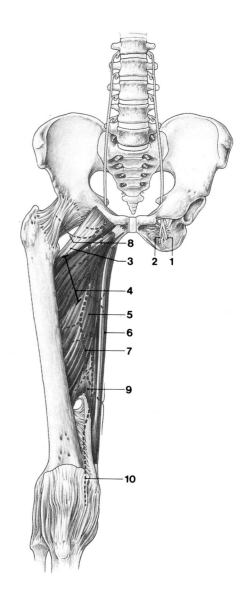

Sciatic nerve block
Anatomy

The sciatic nerve is derived from the lumbosacral trunk (L4-S3). It is the biggest nerve in the body and it emerges from the sciatic foramen at the midpoint between the ischial tuberosity and the greater trochanter.

Indications

The anterior approach is useful for tibial fractures as it can be performed without the patient having to be turned. It can also be used for plastic and orthopaedic procedures of the leg for which, when combined with femoral nerve block, it produces a large area of anaesthesia. Alternatively, a caudal block may be easier to perform if an extensive block is required.

Drugs

1% lidocaine or 1% mepivacaine are suitable for short procedures. 0.25% bupivacaine should be used for longer operations. The volume injected varies with age, from 8ml for a 3 year old child to 20ml for a 12 year old, or 0.5ml.kg^{-1} body weight. The dose regime for brachial plexus

| Age (yrs) | Volume (ml) | | Concentration (%) | |
			L and M	B
0-4	Height (cm)	/12	0.7 - 0.8	0.19
5-8	Height (cm)	/10	0.8 - 0.9	0.25
9-16	Height (cm)	/7	0.9 - 1	0.25

Table 12.Simplified dose regime for sciatic nerve block.
B=Bupivacaine, L=Lidocaine, M=Mepivacaine

block (p. 127) may also be employed for block of the sciatic nerve. Maximum dose levels must be strictly adhered to, particularly when additional nerve blocks, such as femoral, are planned. Adequate volumes are essential to reach the nerves. It can be achieved by diluting the solution when maximum doses have been reached.

Technique
Posterior approach
The sciatic nerve (L4,5, S1,2,3) can be blocked by the posterior approach as it emerges from the sciatic foramen (Fig. 101). The patient may be placed in the lithotomy position, or supine with the leg raised, and the needle is inserted at the midpoint of a line joining the ischial tuberosity and the greater trochanter.

Fig. 101. Posterior sciatic nerve block.

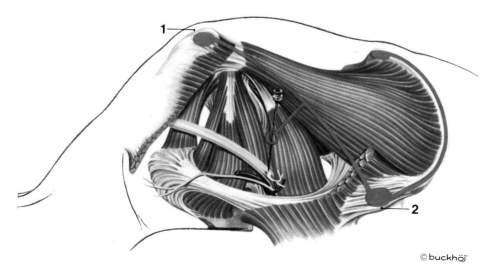

© buckhöj

143

Anterior approach

Alternatively, the anterior approach can be used, and this has been described in children (10). The point of needle insertion is shown in Fig. 102. A 7cm short bevel needle is advanced until it contacts the femur. It is then withdrawn and re-directed medially past the lesser trochanter of the femur. As the needle is passing through the adductor magnus muscle, there is marked resistance to injection, but loss of resistance is felt as the needle emerges from the deep surface of the muscle and pierces the fascia which lies in front of the sciatic nerve. The position of the needle can be confirmed with a nerve stimulator. If the latter is used, the needle should preferably be teflon-coated.

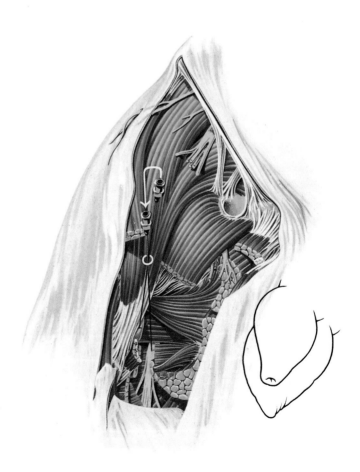

Fig. 102. Anterior sciatic nerve block.

Tibial nerve block

Anatomy

The sciatic nerve divides, at approximately the apex of the popliteal fossa, into the tibial and the common peroneal nerves which supply the calf and peroneal muscles and the area of skin shown in Fig 103.

Indications

These blocks are not commonly performed, but they can be used for surgery within the appropriate areas. Tibial nerve block was developed to reduce gastrocnemius tone in children with extensor spasm resulting from a head injury. While the muscle is relaxed, the foot can be manipulated and plastered at right angles so that the patient can be stood up. This allows more rapid recovery of postural reflexes and assists rehabilitation (11).

Drugs

Depending on the duration of surgery and the age of the child, 1% lidocaine, 1% mepivacaine or 0.25% bupivacaine are used in a dose of 1-5ml.

Technique

These blocks are easily performed by inserting a needle into the popliteal fossa. Loss of resistance is felt as the fascia covering the popliteal fossa is penetrated, and the needle is then advanced a further 5mm.

Fig. 103.

1. Sural nerve
2. Small saphenous vein
3. Medial gastrocnemius muscle
4. Popliteal vein
5. Popliteal artery
6. Medial condyle of femur
7. Tibial nerve
8. Sural artery
9. Lateral gastrocnemius muscle
10. Common peroneal nerve
11. Lateral condyle of femur

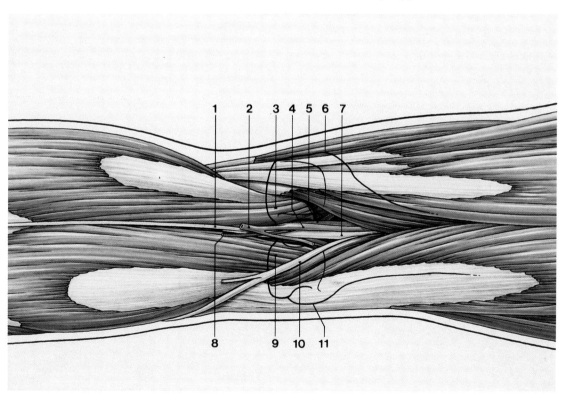

Ankle block

Fig. 104. Ankle block.

1. Saphenous nerve
2. Long saphenous vein
3. Anterior tibial muscle
4. Dep peroneal nerve
5. Extensor hallucis longus muscle
6. Superficial peroneal nerve

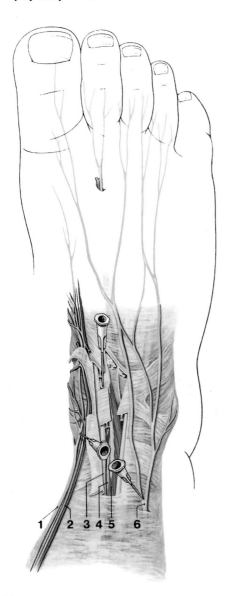

Fig. 104. Ankle block.

1. Saphenous nerve
2. Long saphenous vein
3. Anterior tibial muscle
4. Dep peroneal nerve
5. Extensor hallucis longus muscle
6. Superficial peroneal nerve

Indications

Ankle blocks can be used alone for minor operations in older children or as an adjunct to light general anaesthesia. They are also useful for providing postoperative analgesia following otherwise painful operations such as removal of ingrowing toenails.

Anatomy and technique

Five nerves, the terminal branches of the sciatic and femoral nerves, supply the foot.

Deep peroneal nerve

The anterior tibial (or deep peroneal) nerve, lies deep to the retinaculum which must be penetrated if the nerve is to be anaesthetised. Loss of resistance can be felt as a short-bevel needle pierces it.

Superficial peroneal nerve

The superficial peroneal nerve divides and runs down the anterior aspect of the foot between its midpoint and the lateral malleolus (Fig. 104); the saphenous nerve runs between the midpoint and the medial malleolus. The nerves are blocked by subcutaneous infiltration around these sites.

Drugs

Depending on the duration of surgery and the age of the child, 1% lidocaine, 1% mepivacaine or 0.25% bupivacaine are given in a dose of 1 - 5ml for each nerve to be blocked.

Fig. 105. The cutaneous distribution.

Saphenous nerve

Superficial peroneal nerve

Deep peroneal nerve

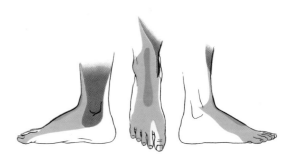

Tibial nerve

The anterior tibial lies immediately lateral to the anterior tibial artery on the dorsum of the foot, and the tibial nerve lies in a space between the medial malleolus and the Achilles tendon (Fig 106). The retinaculum overlying this space can be felt and the needle should be advanced a few millimetres after loss of resistance has been detected. Care should be taken not to inject into the nearby posterior tibial vessels.

Sural nerve

The other three nerves lie subcutaneously and as their superficial landmarks are less well defined, they are blocked by subcutaneous infiltration. The sural nerve runs between the lateral malleolus and the Achilles tendon (Fig 107).

Drugs

Depending on the duration of surgery and the age of the child, 1% lidocaine, 1% mepivacaine or 0.25% bupivacaine are given in a dose of 1-5ml for each nerve to be blocked.

The cutaneous distribution is shown in Fig. 106.

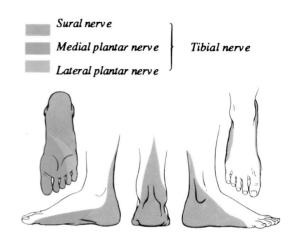

Sural nerve
Medial plantar nerve   } Tibial nerve
Lateral plantar nerve

Fig. 106. The cutaneous distribution.

Fig. 107. Tibial and sural nerve block.

1. Flexor retinaculum
2. Tibial nerve
3. Posterior tibial artery
4. Sural nerve
5. Short saphenous vein

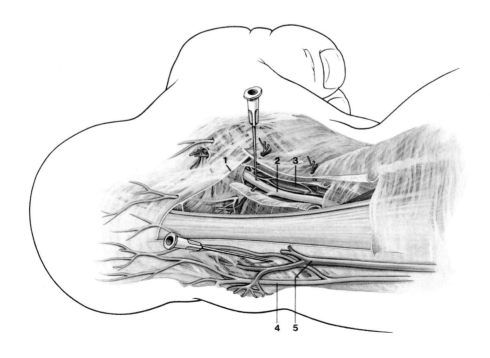

References

1. Cousins MJ & Bridenbaugh PD (1987) Neural Blockade in Clinical Anesthesia and Management of Pain, 2nd Ed. JB Lippincott USA

2. Moore DC (1961) Regional Block. Charles C Thomas, USA

3. Eriksson E (1979) Illustrated Handbook in Local Anaesthesia, 2nd Ed. Schultz Forlag, Copenhagen

4. Raj PP (1985) Handbook of Regional Anesthesia Churchill Livingstone, USA

5. Wildsmith JAW & Armitage EN (1987) (eds). Principles and Practice of Regional Anaesthesia, Churchill Livingstone, Edinburgh, London, Melbourne, New York

6. Khoo ST & Brown TCK (1983) Femoral Nerve Block - The Anatomical Basis for a Single Injection Technique. Anaesth Intens Care 11, 40

7. Winnie AP, Ramamurthy SR, Durrany Z (1973) The Inguinal Perivascular Technique of Lumbar Plexus Anaesthesia: The "3 in 1 block". Anesth Analg (Cleve) 52:989

8. Brown TCK & Dickens DVR: Another Approach to Lateral Cutaneous Nerve of Thigh Block. Anaesth Intens Care 14: 126

9. Brown TCK & Hughes P (1986) Posterior Cutaneous Nerve of Thigh Block. Anaesth Intens Care. In press

10. McNicol LR (1985) Sciatic Nerve Block for Children. Anaesthesia 40:410

11. Kempthorne PM & Brown TCK (1984) Nerve Blocks around the Knee in Children. Anaesth Intens Care 12:14

Intercostal nerve block

Claude Saint-Maurice

After intercostal nerve blocks, local anaesthetic is rapidly absorbed from the surrounding membranes and systemic toxicity can occur if many nerves are blocked. For this reason its use is limited in children over six years old in whom relatively large doses of local anaesthetic are necessary. If more extensive analgesia is required, an other block is more appropriate.

Fig 108. Anatomy of the first and second intercostal nerves.

1. Intercostal nerve (ventral ramus)
2. Muscular branch
3. Lateral cutaneous branch
4. Branch to transversus thoracis muscle
5. Anterior cutaneous branch
6. Endothoracic fascia
7. Posterior intercostal membrane
8. Intercostalis externus muscle
9. Intercostalis internus muscle
10. Intercostalis intimus muscle
11. External intercostal membrane

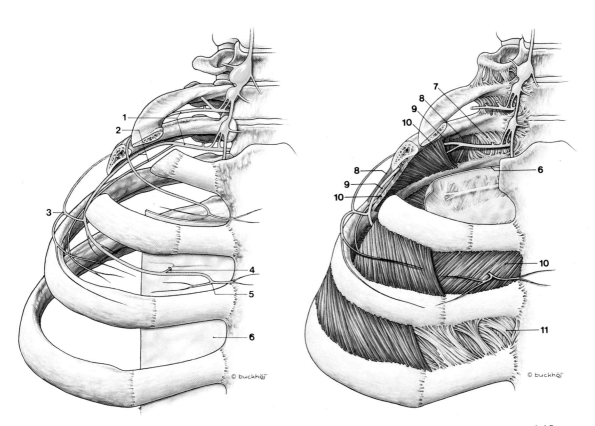

© buckhöj

© buckhöj

Anatomy

After crossing the paravertebral space, the main branch of the intercostal nerve runs with the intercostal blood vessels in the concave subcostal groove. The nerve runs close to the pleura, from which it is separated only by the endothoracic fascia, so there is a high risk of perforating the pleura when a needle is inserted for intercostal nerve block. At the point where the costal angle crosses the posterior axillary line, the nerve is a few millimetres from the inferior edge of the rib exactly beneath the intercostal vessels. (Figs. 108 and 109)

Fig 109. Anatomy of the seventh intercostal nerve.

Indications

If rib resection has not been needed for surgical access (which is usually the case in children), the block may be performed for post-thoracotomy analgesia (1, 2). Blocks can be done, one above and one below the incision, by the anaesthetist at the end of surgery.

Alternatively, the surgeon can give the injections under direct vision before he closes the chest. In both cases, good post-operative analgesia is achieved without attendant respiratory problems.

Intercostal block is also indicated to relieve the pain of fractured ribs. It should not be used if more than three ribs are affected since multiple blocks may produce high blood levels of local

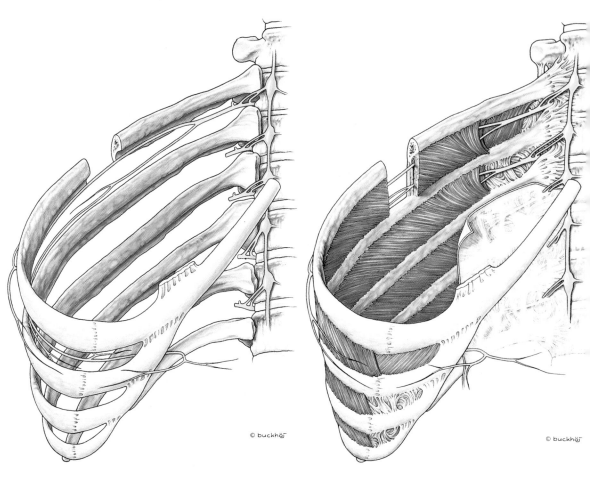

© buckhöj
© buckhöj

150

anaesthetic. The pain relief not only improves the comfort of the child, but also prevents hypoventilation due to pain (3). Although this improvement in ventilation is only transitory, continuous intercostal block is not advisable.

Intercostal blocks cannot be justified for analgesia of the abdominal wall since this can be achieved better and more safely with an epidural. With the latter, there is no risk of perforating a distended viscus, as may happen when a lower intercostal block is being attempted. Severe contralateral lung disease is also a contra-indication because even a small pneumothorax on the healthy side, caused by accidental pleural puncture, may leave the patient dangerously compromised.

Drugs and doses

The two drugs most commonly used are lidocaine 0.5%, which gives about two hours analgesia, and bupivacaine 0.25% which gives 3 to 4 hours. The addition of adrenaline 1 in 200.000 doubles the duration of the block.

One to three ml of local anaesthetic is needed, according to the age of the child, for each intercostal space. It is dangerous to use more concentrated solutions or larger volumes because of the risk of overdosage. For the same reason, a continuous catheter technique is not recommended, and no more than four intercostal nerves should be blocked. However, Schulte Steinberg

and the present author have used 0.166% bupivacaine with success, and with this low concentration, it is possible to block several nerves. The solution is prepared by adding one volume of saline to two volumes of bupivacaine 0.25%.

The total dose of bupivacaine should not exceed $2mg.kg^{-1}$. Absorption of local anaesthetic from the intercostal space is rapid in adults and even more so in children, and the volume of distribution and the clearance are greater than in adults. Moreover, there is a relationship between the haematocrit and whole blood and plasma concentrations of local anaesthetic (4, 5 and Table 13).

In the adult, a solution of preservative-free morphine $0.5mg.ml^{-1}$ has been given with bupivacaine $0.25mg.ml^{-1}$ and this provides analgesia of long duration (6). However, the morphine content seems too high for safe use in children.

Technique

As for any regional technique, an intravenous infusion is set up before the block. Adult patients are often placed in the supine position (7, 8), but for a child, the lateral position is best with the side to be blocked uppermost and the arm placed on the head so that the scapula is drawn upwards and, as far as possible, clear of the ribs. This happens to be the position often chosen for thoracic surgery.

Fig. 110. Intercostal nerve block technique.

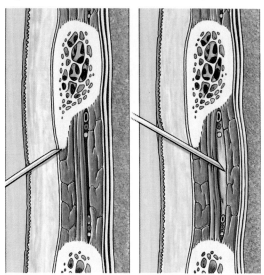

Table 13. Effect of hematocrit on whole blood/plasma concentration ratio ( ). Rothstein P et al (1986) Anesth Analg 65:625.

		Bupivacaine base µg/ml		
Patient	Hematocrit	Whole blood	Plasma	
1	32	2.13	2.71	0.79
2	35	2.07	2.67	0.78
3	30	1.86	2.28	0.82
4	39	1.23	1.85	0.66
5	33	1.47	1.80	0.82
6	34	1.71	2.52	0.68
7	50	1.84	2.95	0.62
8	59	1.76	2.88	0.61
9	50	1.23	2.62	0.47
10	49	1.88	2.45	0.77
11	53	1.74	2.84	0.61

Skin preparation should be as meticulous as for a spinal or epidural. The inferior border of the rib is located three to five cm from the posterior midline. A 24 or 25G, 30mm needle is selected and the skin is punctured at this point. The needle is advanced upwards, at an angle of 120° to the skin, towards the lower border of the rib (Fig 111). It is important that the syringe should be attached to the needle to mimimise the effects of a pneumothorax in the case of perfora-tion of the pleura. As soon as bony contact has been made, the needle is withdrawn about 2mm clear of the rib and the angle is reduced to 60°, the second finger of the left hand pushing down the skin so that the needle is now pointing slightly downwards. It is then advanced 3 to 4mm so that it passes beneath the rib, with the bevel facing cephalad. This whole procedure can also be performed with a 25G percutaneous cannula.

After an aspiration test for air and blood to exclude puncture of the pleura or a blood vessel, the local anaesthetic is injected. If fresh bony contact is made during the course of the injection, it is advisable to start again by making the skin puncture site slightly more inferior. Analgesia is demonstrable in less than ten minutes.

In the above description, the puncture site is 3 to 5cm from the posterior midline and since the ribs are often covered at this point by the paravertebral muscles, they are not felt as easily as in the posterior axillary line. However, the latter landmark can only be used for the lower ribs as it is often crossed by the surgical incision.

Complications

Pneumothorax due to perforation of the pleura is the obvious risk, though the effects can be minimised by the use of small needles (24 to 27G). If this complication is suspected, the child must be kept under close clinical observation. More than one chest radiograph may be needed to demonstrate a pneumothorax.

Puncture of one of the intercostal vessels is possible, but is not serious unless it is overlooked or ignored.

Overdosage is the most important complication because of the rapid absorption of local anaesthetic which follows intercostal blocks. It is this factor which limits the usefulness of, and indications for, the technique (7, 8).

If the anaesthetist adheres to the indications mentioned above, intercostal block is a safe and useful, if somewhat limited, technique, but severe systemic toxicity will result if more is asked of it than it can safely give.

References

1. Cronin KD, Davis MJ (1976) Intercostal block for post-operative pain relief. Anesth Intensive Care 4
2. Delmot F, Murphy MB (1983) Intercostal nerve blockade for fracture ribs and post-operative analgesia. Regional Anesthesia 151
3. Faust RJ, Nauss LA (1976) Post-thoracotomy intercostal block. Comparison of its effects on pulmonary function with those of intramuscular méperidine. Anesth Analg Curr Res 54
4. Rothstein P, Arthur GR, Feldman H, Barash PG, Kopf G, Sudan N, Covino BG (1982) Pharmacokinetics of bupivacaine in children following intercostal block. Anesthesiology 57
5. Rothstein P, Arthur GR, Feldman HS, Kopf GS, Covino BG (1986) Bupivacaine for intercostal nerve blocks in children. Anesth Analg 65
6. Lecron L, Bogaerts J, Lafont N, Balatoni E (1983) Utilisation des morphiniques dans les blocs nerveux périphériques - "L'anesthésie devant le problème de la douleur". Ars Medici Bruxelles 1
7. Lecron L (1986) Anesthésie des nerfs intercostaux in Anesthésie Loco-Régionale. Arnette Edit Paris 349
8. Moore DC (1962) Intercostal nerve blocking: 4333 patients: indications, technique and complications. Anesth Analg 41

Intrapleural regional anaesthesia

Claude Saint-Maurice

Intrapleural regional anaesthesia was described for the first time by Kvalheim and Reiestad in 1984 (1), Mc Ilvaine et al used this technique in children in 1988 (2).

Indications
It can be used for upper abdominal procedures and for thoracotomies.

Contraindications
Intrapleural blood or fluid is a contraindication because this dilutes the local anaesthetic solution and may reduce its effectiveness. If the pleura is inflamed absorption of local anaesthetic is rapid and toxic concentrations may be reached. A bupivacaine concentration of 4.9µg.ml^{-1} was measured five minutes following injection of a 0.5% bupivacaine solution (5). Contralateral pneumothorax is a contraindication for obvious reasons.

Drugs and doses
Bupivacaine in concentrations of 0.25%, 0.375% and 0.5% is the only local anaesthetic to have been used. In adults Reiestad and colleagues (3) demonstrated that with 20 ml of 0.5% solution Cmax reached 1.18 µg.ml^{-1} (range 0.39-1.54) and was reached in 20 minutes. In a study which included only adults, Seltzer and colleagues used 30 ml of 0.5% solution with 1:100.000 adrenaline (5). The maximal concentrations was 3.27 µg.ml^{-1} (Table 14) a high value which might produce neurological signs.

Rosenberg and colleagues (4) have used a continuous infusion of bupivacaine. An initial injection of 15 to 20 ml of 0.5% bupivacaine was given, depending on the patient's weight. One hour later a continuous infusion of 0.25% bupivacaine was started, and eventually produced plasma concentrations which could be regarded as potentially toxic.

Patient	Cmax (µg/ml)	Tmax (min)
1	2.42	15
2	2.05	30
3	1.71	15
4	1.58	30
5	2.23	15
6	1.10	30
7	1.86	30
8	3.27	10
9	2.23	15
10	2.25	15
Mean± SD	2.07 ±0.58	20.5 ± 8.3

Table 14. Maximum plasma bupivacaine concentration (Cmax) and time when these levels were measured (Tmax).

Similar results have been obtained in children by McIlvaine who used 0.25% bupivacaine solution with 1:200.000 adrenaline (2). The children in this series also received intravenous diazepam, rectal chloral hydrate and rectal acetaminophen if pyrexia was present. The nurse was allowed to increase the infusion rate incrementally to a maximum of 1 ml.kg^{-1}·h^{-1} to obtain adequate analgesia. In 5 of the 14 children the plasma concentration exceeded 4 µg.ml^{-1} and in 1 it exceeded 7 µg.ml^{-1}. The conclusion is obvious. Continous infusion, at least when administered by this regimen, results in dangerous drug accumulation.

Technique
In adults the anaesthetist inserts the intrapleural catheter through a 16G Tuohy needle at the 8th intercostal space, 10 cm from the midline, with the patient in the lateral position. When the needle enters the pleural space, the plunger of the syringe is sucked forward because of the negative intrapleural pressure. The needle is introduced at an angle of 30° in the middle of the intercostal space to avoid damage to veins and nerves.

Alternatively the block can be performed by the surgeon before chest closure. A 20G catheter is introduced through a 18G Tuohy needle imme-

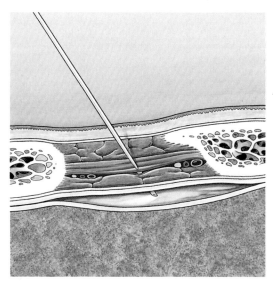

Fig. 111. Intrapleural technique.

diately below the intercostal space. The catheter is fixed to the chest and a sterile plastic dressing applied. The continuous infusion is started when the patient has regained consciousness.

Conclusion
The results of intrapleural regional anaesthesia, in terms of postoperative analgesia, may be attractive, but the plasma concentrations of bupivacaine are unacceptably high. More investigations are necessary before the potential of this technique can be established in children.

References
1. Kvalheim L, Reiestad F (1984) Interpleural catheter in the management of postoperative pain. Anesthesiology 61, 3A: A231
2. Mc Ilvaine WB, Knox RF, Fennessey PV, Goldstein M (1988) Continuous infusion of bupivacaine via intrapleural catheter for analgesia after thoracotomy in children. Anesthesiology 69:261
3. Reiestad F, Stroskag KE, Holmqvist E (1986) Intrapleural administration of bupivacaine in postoperative management of pain. Anesthesiology 65, 3A: A 204
4. Rosenberg PH, Scheinin BMA, Lepantalo MJ, Lindfors O (1987) Continuous intrapleural infusion of bupivacaine for analgesia after thoracotomy. Anesthesiology 67:811
5. Seltzer JL, Larijani GE, Goldberg ME, Marr AT (1987) Intrapleural bupivacaine, A kinetic and dynamic evaluation. Anesthesiology 67:798

Ilioinguinal and iliohypogastric nerve block

Ottheinz Schulte Steinberg

Anatomy

These nerves are formed by branches which arise from the spinal cord at the level of T12 and L1. After tracking laterally and forwards, they pierce the internal oblique muscle at a point just below and 1 to 2cm medial to the anterior iliac spine and they both lie between the muscle and the aponeurosis of the external oblique (Fig. 112). The nerves supply the skin of the lower abdomen and the inguinal region.

Fig. 112.

1. *External oblique muscle*
2. *Internal oblique muscle*
3. *Anterior superior iliac spine*
4. *Transversus abdominis muscle*
5. *Ilioinguinal nerve*
6. *Inguinal ligament*
7. *Iliohypogastric nerve*
8. *Genital branch of the genitofemoral nerve*
9. *Spermatic cord*
10. *Pubic tubercle*
11. *Superficial inguinal ring*
12. *Inguinal hernia*

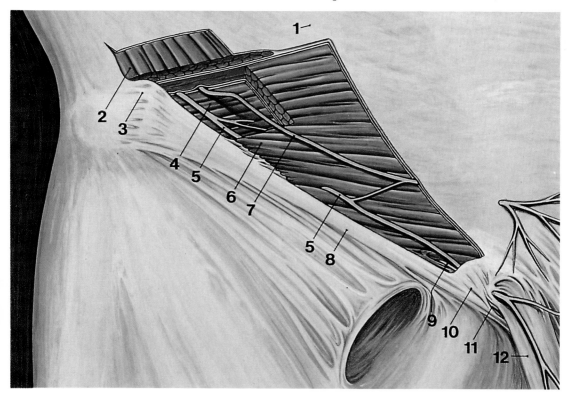

Indications

The block is used for postoperative analgesia for inguinal surgery, such as herniotomy and orchidopexy. It is important to realise that it provides skin analgesia only. However, when used as an adjunct to general anaesthesia, it enables the latter to be maintained at a light level. If the block is to be used for surgery without any general anaesthesia, it is necessary to infiltrate the hernial sac; the line of the skin incision may also require infiltration.

Contraindications

There are no special contraindications

Drugs and dosage

Bupivacaine 0.5% is the drug of choice. It is given in a dose of 0,25 mg.kg^{-1}.

Technique

A 20G, short bevel needle is inserted just below and medial to the anterior superior iliac spine. The distance medial depends on the size of the child, being 0.5cm in the infant and 2cm in the adolescent. The needle is slowly advanced until there is a loss of resistance, which occurs as the aponeurosis of the external oblique is pierced. The needle is then immobilised in this position. An aspiration test is carried out and, if it is negative, local anaesthetic is injected from a 10ml syringe. The drug spreads in the layer between the internal oblique and the external oblique aponeurosis, and comes into contact with both nerves. For bilateral procedures, the same technique is performed on the other side.

Complications

The block is very safe, but, as with almost all other regional techniques, it is possible to inject the local anaesthetic intravascularly.
Careful aspiration before (and if necessary repeated aspiration during) injection should ensure that this does not happen.

If the needle is too long or is inserted too deeply, an intraperitoneal injection may be accidentally given. Absorption will then be rapid and toxic plasma concentrations may be reached.

Summary

Ilio-inguinal and hypogastric block provides skin analgesia after inguinal surgery. It requires smaller quantities of drug than a caudal and does not cause significant motor block. However, unless it is supplemented with local infiltration of the hernial sac and the line of the skin incision, it is not adequate for operative surgery of the inguinal canal.

References

1. Brown TCK, Schulte Steinberg O (1988) Neural Blockade. Ed. by Cousins MJ, Bridenbaugh PO, 2nd ed. JB Lippincott Co, Philadelphia
2. Scott DB (1989) Techniques of Regional Anaesthesia, Mediglobe, Fribourg

Penile block

Jean-Luc Hody

For many generations, the operation of circumcision has been performed on healthy children for reasons of religion, ritual or hygiene. Early, crude attempts to render the foreskin insensitive included the application of cold, prior induction of ischaemia by mechanical means and even psychological conditioning of older children ("to achieve manhood"). Operations on the foreskin and penis, as for the treatment of hypo-spadias, and circumcision for surgical reasons, are of much more recent origin.

General anaesthesia has paved the way for better controlled and less traumatic surgery, but at a price. Deep levels of anaesthesia are required, and the problem of post-operative pain remains unsolved. As a result, the restless, distressed child may pull off his dressings and increase the chances of infection and haemorrhage.

Regional techniques, such as spinal, peridural and, more particularly, caudal block, have made it possible to eliminate these disadvantages, but some expertise is required to perform them and, since they act over a wide area, they exert unwanted side-effects. Penile block is an attractive alternative because it does not call for great skill and it provides excellent analgesia during and after the operation. It also confers physiological benefit. In a recent study, (1) heart rate and blood pressure remained stable at the time of circumcision in those neonates who had received a penile block, whereas these parameters increased significantly in unanaesthetised babies. Furthermore, oxygen saturation, which decreased by as much as 22% in the unanaesthetised group, fell by only about 10% in the penile block group.

Anatomy

The penis receives its innervation from the right and left dorsal nerves of the penis. These originate from the roots of the pudendal plexus, which is formed by the 2nd-4th sacral nerves.

Internal pudendal nerve

The internal pudendal nerve is the terminal branch of the pudendal plexus and is formed mainly by the 2nd and 3rd sacral roots. It divides into two branches:

Perineal nerve

The perineal nerve, consists of a superficial branch innervating the skin over the anterior part of the perineum, the scrotum and the underside of the penis, and a deep or musculo-urethral branch, containing both motor and sensory fibres and supplying the bulbus urethrae, urethra and base of the glans.

Dorsal nerve of the penis

The dorsal nerve of the penis is contained within the same sheath as the internal pudendal vessels and lies deep to the suspensory ligament of the penis. A few millimetres after passing under the symphysis, it sends out small ramifications to the lower part of the penis and the frenulum. Distally, it becomes superficial and innervates the dorsal surface of the penis and the glans. The two dorsal nerves, with the deep dorsal vein and the two dorsal arteries, are enclosed in a compartment bounded externally by Buck's fascia.

It should be noted that the internal pudendal nerve consists of somatic fibres, innervating the skin and some of the muscles of the perineum, sympathetic fibres coming from the communicating sacral branches, and parasympathetic fibres originating from the sacral parasympathetic outflow.

It should also be pointed out that the skin at the base of the penis is innervated by the ilio-inguinal nerve (L1) and occasionally by a branch of the genito-femoral nerve (L1-2).

Complications

It is essential that adrenaline is not used because of the danger of ischaemia. Haematoma and IV injection are other possible complications.

Technique

After a suitable premedication, light general anaesthesia, O_2, N_2O and halothane, or ketamine (Ketalar) is induced so that the child is unresponsive and immobile when the needle is being inserted and the local anaesthetic injected. Strict asepsis is observed and the injection is prepared beforehand. 0.5% bupivacaine **without** adrenaline is used in a dose of 1mg.kg^{-1}. A short (15mm) 25G needle can be used, although some authors use a 23G (2) or a 27G (3) needle.

With the penis slightly extended, the symphysis pubis is palpated at the junction between the penis and the inferior end of the anterior abdominal wall. As the palpating finger moves inferiorly, a difference can be felt between the anterior abdominal wall, which is infiltrated with fat, and Buck's fascia over the root of the penis, which is free of fat. Some workers give two lateral injections (4,5) whereas others (2,6) retract the superficial dorsal vein of the penis and give a single injection in the midline. It is unnecessary to make contact with the symphysis or to seek paraesthesiae, the sole aim being to pierce the fascia. A click may sometimes be felt when this has occurred. The injected local anaesthetic spreads to left and right and anaes-thetises both the deep nerves. The superficial nerves are anaesthetised by withdrawing the needle superficial to Buck's fascia and injecting solution subcutaneously to left and right (Fig. 113). Occasionally, a midline septum exists and prevents bilateral spread of the solution. A second injection must then be performed on the unanaesthetised side.

Conclusion

The great advantages of penile block are that it is relatively easy to perform compared with other techniques, it results in less vomiting (7) no post-operative pain and, hence, minimal post-operative analgesic requirements (8,9,10) and it does not cause retention of urine (6,7). For these reasons, it has a very important role in outpatient treatment and day-stay surgery.

Fig. 113. Penile block technique.

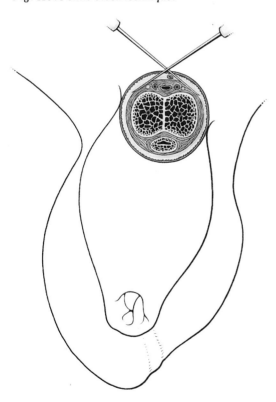

References

1. Maxwell LG, Yaster M, Wetzel RC (1986) Penile nerve block reduces the physiologic stress of newborn circumcision. Anesthesiology 65:3A:432
2. Armitage EN (1985) Block of dorsal nerves of penis (penile block). Regional anaesthesia in paediatrics. Clinics in Anaesthesiology Vol 3 no 3
3. Kirya C, Werthmann MW (1978) Neonatal circumcision and penile dorsal nerve block - a painless procedure. J Pediatr 92:998
4. Defalque R (1983) Simplified penile block. Regional anaesthesia 8:45
5. Goulding F (1981) Penile block for postoperative pain relief in penile surgery. J Urol 126:337
6. Van Zundert A (1985) Penile dorsal nerve block. Acta Anaesth Belg 36:41
7. Yeoman P, Cooke R, Hain W (1983) Penile block for circumcision Anaesthesia 38:862
8. Tozbikian K (1983) Postoperative penile block. Simple, safe, effective. Anaesthesiology Topics 2,7
9. Rodrigo M, Ong L, Waheed A (1984) Dorsal nerve block of penis in Chinese children. Brit J Anaesth 56:934
10. White J, Harrison B, Richmond P, Procter A, Curran J (1983) Postoperative analgesia for circumcision. Brit Med J 286:1934

Intravenous regional anaesthesia

Ottheinz Schulte Steinberg

Indications

Intravenous regional anaesthesia (IVRA) can be used for certain operations on the arms and legs. In general, the technique is more suitable for superficial and distal procedures than for deep and proximal ones, though it is possible to reduce fractures of the radius and ulna under IVRA (1).

Contraindications

It is unsuitable for long operations during which normal tourniquet time might be exceeded and in which tourniquet pain may become a problem. It is also contraindicated for procedures in which meticulous haemostasis is required and in which the surgeon cannot rely on postoperative pressure dressings for the control of bleeding. It is not practical to use IVRA for operations on the upper arm or the thigh because the tourniquet inevitably encroaches on, and may obscure, the operating field.

Drugs

Lidocaine 0.25%-0.5% has been used successfully for several years, but prilocaine, in the same concentration and in a dose of 3mg.kg^{-1}, is the drug of choice. This is because prilocaine is taken up in significant amounts in the lung so, in the event of the drug accidentally leaking past the cuff, it is unlikely that high concentrations of prilocaine will reach the left side of the heart and enter the systemic circula-tion. However, as pointed out in the chapter on Pharmacology and Pharmacokinetics, prilocaine is best avoided in infants because of methaemo-globinaemia. Accidents have been reported following the use of bupivacaine, for which no such protective mechanism operates, and this agent is therefore contraindicated.

Equipment

For intravenous access, a plastic cannula is preferred since it is less likely to cut out of the vein than a needle. Reliable, regularly-serviced pneumatic tourniquets should be available in more than one size, preferably with the double cuff system. Comparatively large volumes of local anaesthetic are required so 20ml is the most suitable syringe size.

Technique

IVRA can easily be performed by an anaesthetist who has no knowledge of other regional techniques. Although this may appear at first sight to be an advantage, it may also be the reason why accidents have occured. Insertion of the plastic intravenous cannula in the periphery of the limb is the key to success. The limb is exsanguinated by elevation and by simultaneous digital occlusion of the arterial supply for a period of three minutes. Painless exsanguination of fractured limbs may also be achieved by using pneumatic splints. (2)

Alternatively, an Esmarch bandage can be applied. The tourniquet is then placed round the upper part of the limb and inflated to a pressure of 100 torr above normal arterial pressure. Higher pressures have been used - Carrell and Eyring (3) originally suggested 180-240 torr for the arm and 350-500 torr for the leg.

When a double-cuff tourniquet is being used, the proximal cuff should be inflated first. Local anaesthetic is then injected slowly through the peripherally-placed plastic cannula. The distal cuff is inflated when analgesia has extended right up to the proximal cuff. 5 to 7 minutes is usually required for this. The proximal cuff is then released. However, the distal cuff should remain inflated for at least 20 minutes even if the operation has been completed within a shorter time. This is to give adequate opportunity for the local anaesthetic solution to become bound to tissues. If the tourniquet is released before this has happened, a large amount of drug may suddenly enter the circulation and produce toxic effects (4).

Complications

The main complication of intravenous regional anaesthesia is tourniquet cuff failure which may result in high plasma concentrations of local anaesthetic and systemic toxicity. However, studies in adults have shown that rapid injection can produce intravenous pressure higher than tourniquet pressure. This can cause the drug to leak into the circulation even when the cuff is functioning perfectly. There is also the possibility that leakage can occur through intra-osseous vascular channels (5) which are protected from tourniquet pressure by the surrounding bone.

The anaesthetist should therefore be constantly alert for signs of systemic toxicity and should be ready to treat the cardiopulmonary collapse which may follow.

Conclusion

Intravenous regional anaesthesia is a useful technique, but it usually requires general anaesthesia for children below the age of 7 years. For older children, sedation is helpful.

References

1. Tucker GL, Batten JB, Hjort D, Ross ERS et al (1986) Intravenous regional anaesthesia for the treatment of upper limb injuries in childhood. Aust NZ J Surg 56:153
2. Rose RJ (1987) Use of an air splint to provide limb exsanguination during intravenous regional anaesthesia in children. Regional anesthesia 12:8.
3. Carrell, E.D. and Eyring, E.J (1971) Intravenous regional anesthesia for childhood fractures. Trauma 11:301
4. Rosenberg PH, Kalso EA, Tuominen MK and Lindèn HB (1983) Acute bupivacaine toxicity a result of venous leakage under the tourniquet cuff during Bier block. Anesthesiology 58:95
5. Robson CH (1936) Anesthesia in children. Am J Surg 34:468

Topical anaesthesia

Ottheinz Schulte Steinberg

Indications
Topical anaesthesia in children is mainly used on the mucosal surfaces of the pharynx and airway to facilitate endotracheal intubation, and for bronchoscopy.

Contraindications
The technique should not be applied to infected membranes.

Drugs and dosage
Lidocaine without adrenaline is used. Concentrations of 0.5%, 1% and 2% may be used depending on the age of the child, the lower concentrations being more suitable for infants. 3mg.kg^{-1} body weight has been suggested as the maximum safe dose of plain lidocaine in an adult (1). However, the appearance of toxic effects depends almost as much on the site of injection as on the dose, and also upon the rate of absorption of the drug. Absorption from mucous membranes is very rapid and can produce plasma concentrations comparable with those resulting from intravenous injection (2). For topical anaesthesia, therefore, it is probably wise to limit the dose to 1.5mg.kg^{-1}.

Technique
A 2ml syringe is filled with the calculated amount of lidocaine appropriate for the size of the child. A piece of blind-ending tubing with several small side-holes is attached. After the induction of general anaesthesia, minute quantities of local anaesthetic are instilled in increments as the tubing is inserted through the nose, over the back of the tongue and into the pharynx. Further instillations are applied to the vocal cords for intubation and to the bronchial tree for bronchoscopy. It is most important to observe the quan-

tity of topical local anaesthetic used and to include it in the calculation of the total amount given if a regional block is also to be performed.

Advantages
In cases where muscle relaxants are contraindicated, topical anaesthesia of the airway facilitates intubation and enables it to be performed relatively quickly without submitting the child to deep general anaesthesia.

Fig. 114. Application of topical anaesthetic to the pharynx.

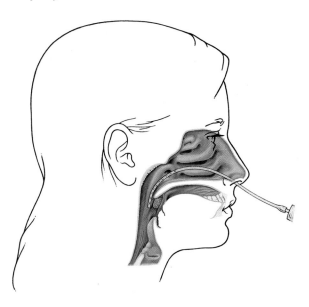

Complications

Overdosage is probably the only important complication, but it is unfortunately very easily achieved. The lowest appropriate concentration should therefore be used, and the commercially available, highly concentrated solutions should be avoided.

References

1. Kelton DA, Daly M, Cooper PD and Canu AW (1970) Plasma lidocaine concentrations following topical aerosal application to the trachea and bronchi. Can Anesth Soc J 17
2. Eyres RL, Kidd J, Oppenheimer RC and Brown TCK (1978) Local anaesthetic plasma levels in children. Anaesth Intens Care 6

Fig. 115. Application of topical anaesthetic to the vocal cords.

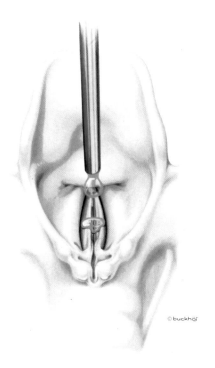

Transcutaneous anaesthesia

Claude Saint-Maurice

The pain caused by a needle prick and the defensive response to this pain are the main reasons why venous cannulation in children can be difficult. The concept of inducing cutaneous anaesthesia by applying local anaesthetic to the skin is not new, but skin is impermeable to the basic, unionised form of the drug responsible for its penetration and diffusion in tissues, and attempts to increase the total unionised content by increasing the concentration were unsuccess-ful. Alcoholic solutions diffuse rapidly in mucous membranes, but do not penetrate skin. An aqueous solution is required but unfortunately the unionised, basic form of local anaesthetics is poorly soluble in water. The solubility is improved in an oil-in-water emulsion, but even then, only 20% of the base can be contained in droplet form and this is insufficient for skin penetration.

Fig. 117.
1. Uptake of local anaesthetic
2. Hydrated straum corneum
3. EMLA Cream
4. Occlusive foil

Recently it has been discovered that when equal quantities of lidocaine and prilocaine are mixed, they melt to form an oil. The melting point of this mixture is 18°C though the melting points of both the individual drugs are much higher. Substances which behave in this way are said to form a eutectic mixture (1). When this oil is used in an emulsion, the proportion of anaesthetic base in a droplet increases four times, to 80%. This is sufficient to penetrate intact skin (Fig 116) even though the concentrations of both lidocaine and prilocaine in the mixture are only 5%. The commercial preparation of lidocaine and prilocaine is known as EMLA - eutectic mixture of local anaesthetics.

Painful cutaneous sensation resulting from mechanical stimuli are transmitted by the fast, myelinated A type fibres and by the slow, unmyelinated C fibres. The latter fibres are also present in the blood vessel wall.

Tolerance

The cream is well tolerated by the skin. Pallor is usually seen when the cream has been applied for an hour or so, and this generally can be taken as a sign of good anaesthesia. Hyperaemia occasionally occurs. The cream should be applied 60 minutes before venepuncture (2).

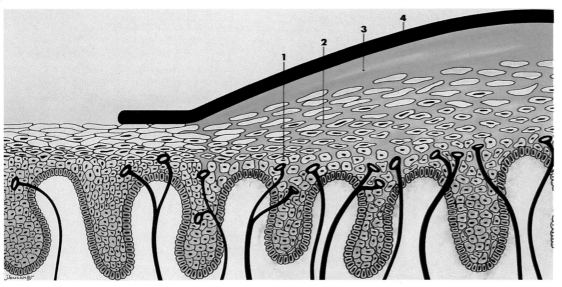

Plasma concentrations

In a study of 22 children aged 3 to 12 months, Engberg (3) applied 2ml of EMLA cream and found that in every case the lidocaine and prilocaine concentrations were less than $0.2\mu g.ml^{-1}$ - a figure which is 25 times smaller than the toxic plasma concentrations. The maximum concentration found for lidocaine was $0.155\mu g.ml^{-1}$ and that for prilocaine was $0.131\mu g.ml^{-1}$. The values for prilocaine were always less than those for lidocaine. An increase of 1.2% in the blood methaemoglobin level has been observed, but no clinical symptoms or signs have been noted.

Directions for use

1 to 1.5ml of the cream is applied thickly to the skin and covered with a transparent occlusive dressing for at least an hour. The dressing is then removed and the skin cleaned with alcohol. Good quality analgesia will last for at least 1 hour after a one hour application. A two hour application will result in 90 minutes of analgesia.

EMLA cream permits painless skin puncture, but it is obviously not effective outside the area of application. Therefore, the anaesthetist must predetermine the site at his preoperative visit, mark it and point it out to the nurse so that the cream is applied to the correct area.

Fig. 117. EMLA cream application.

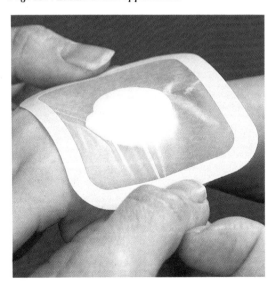

Indications

EMLA can be helpful not only for the intravenous induction of anaesthesia in theatre, but also on the ward when intravenous access is required. It has been used as the sole anaesthetic for minor surgery involving the skin (4-5), and for anaesthesia at the puncture site when a regional block is to be performed.

Contraindications

It is contraindicated in children taking methaemoglobin- producing drugs such as sulphonamides, nitrites or nitrates (6). It is probably unwise to use it in infants less than three months old. The dose should not exceed 5g and the duration of application should not be more than two hours.

Complications

The author is aware of only one case of methaemoglobinaemia. This occurred in a 12 week old infant to whom 5g was applied over a five hour period at two different sites. The child was also receiving a trimethoprim-sulpha-methoxazole mixture. It was treated with methylene blue.

References

1. Evers H, von Dardel O, Juhlin L, Olsen L, Vinnars E (1985) Dermal effects of compositions based on the eutectic mixture of lignocaine and prilocaine. Br J Anaesth 57:997
2. Hallén B, Olsson GL, Uppfeld T (1984) Pain free venepuncture. Anaesthesia 39:369
3. Engberg G, Danielsson K, Henneberg S, Nilsson A (1986) Plasma concentrations of prilocaine and methemoglobin formation in infants after dermal application of a 5% lidocaine, prilocaine cream (EMLA). VIi European Congress of Anaesthesiology Vienna - Abstract 806.
4. Juhlin L, Evers H, Broberg FA (1980) Lidocaine-prilocaine cream for superficial skin surgery and painful lesions. Acta Der Venereol (Stockh) 60:544
5. Lubens HM, Ausden-Moor RW, Shafer AD, Peele RM (1974) Anesthetic patch for painful procedures such as minor operations. Am J Dis Child 128:192
6. Jakobson B, Nilsson A (1985) Methaemoglobinemia associated with a prilocaine, lidocaine cream and trimetroprim sulpha-methaxazole. A case report. Acta Anaesth Scand 29:453

III Pain Management

Post-operative analgesia

Isabelle Murat

The recent interest in regional anaesthesia for children arises chiefly from the fact that it can provide excellent post-operative analgesia. Post-operative pain has traditionally been neglected for two main reasons. Firstly, the assessment of pain is difficult, especially in very young children (1, 2, 3) and, secondly, very few analgesic drugs are completely suitable for use in children. Parenteral opiates have important side-effects and other preparations are either contra-indicated in small babies (4) or are ineffective. This unsatisfactory situation has led some anaesthetists to evade the issue and to claim that the neonate does not feel pain and that therefore no post-operative analgesia is necessary.

Regional techniques are free from the disadvantages of the parenteral opiates. Caudal block was the first to become popular and was found to be safe and effective after circumcision (5), but a variety of techniques are now widely used after major and minor surgery.

Advantages and indications

Outpatient surgery

Regional anaesthesia is usually combined with general anaesthesia. Since minimal amounts of the latter are required, recovery is rapid and post-operative morbidity, particularly nausea and vomiting, is reduced (6, 7). Alternatively, the operation may be performed under general anaesthesia alone and the block inserted at the end. Although recovery time is not so rapid, the analgesia lasts longer.

All regional techniques can provide analgesia which lasts for several hours and reduces post-operative stress (8, 9). Better analgesia is obtained than with parenteral opiates and side-effects are fewer and less severe (9, 10, 11, 12).

For the child undergoing outpatient surgery, it is important that the post-operative course is uneventful and that normal activity returns rapidly, so the regional technique itself should not give rise to undesirable side-effects. Unwanted motor block (9) and retention of urine are possible complications of caudal block which are unpleasant for the child and may delay his discharge from hospital, but they can both be avoided if the appropriate type and concentration of drug and the correct technique are selected.

It is sometimes suggested that regional techniques take a long time to perform and that they are therefore unsuitable for outpatient surgery. In fact, this is untrue, and most of the commonly used techniques can be performed in a relatively short time by the experienced anaesthetist (13).

Major surgery
Although the provision of post-operative pain control is the main objective of regional anaesthesia, other benefits can be expected (14, 15).

Reduction in the stress response
This can be demonstrated in adults after appropriate neural blockade (16, 17), although there is debate as to whether the abolition of the stress response or the stress response itself is the more beneficial. However, in certain at-risk groups, such as young children in poor nutritional condition, abolition of the stress response can be de-

Fig. 118. Effects of epidural anaesthesia. Cortisol response following urinary surgery in children

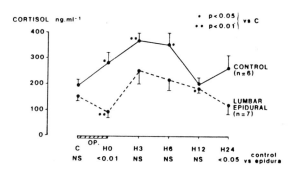

166

sirable because it encourages positive nitrogen balance in the early post-operative period (18) (Fig. 118).

Avoidance of narcotics

This decreases, especially during prolonged surgery, the severity and frequency of undesirable side-effects of these drugs often seen in the post-operative period. Respiratory depression, nausea, vomiting and reduction of gastro-intestinal motility are the most important side-effects and Koren and colleagues (19) have shown that there is wide variation in response to the infusion of morphine in neonates and small babies. The same workers also observed a lower elimination rate for morphine in the newborn.

Reduction in chest complications

It is still a matter for debate whether there is a reduction in chest complications as a result of epidural analgesia. In adults, spirometric para-meters and blood gases can be improved, but the incidence of chest complications in at-risk popul-ations remains high (20, 21, 22). However, epi-dural analgesia is recommended in these patients because it renders physiotherapy easier to tolerate and more effective. Meignier (23) recently con-firmed these findings in children with respiratory disabilities who received post-operative thoracic epidural block.

Other benefits

Improved blood flow to areas affected by the block and reduced incidence of deep vein throm-bosis are less important in children than in adults. The incidence of deep vein thrombosis in children is very low indeed.

Indications

The indications for regional anaesthesia can be considered now that the advantages have been defined.

1. Major orthopaedic surgery is often painful because of the need for physiotherapy afterwards. In some conditions, such as limb lengthening procedures in children, traction on the limb is increased at intervals in the first few days after operation and epidural analgesia is invaluable for rendering these manipulations painless. It is particularly important that ischaemia does not occur after orthopaedic surgery if a child is re-ceiving epidural analgesia since the ischaemia will be painless and may go unreported. The colour, temperature and motor function of the legs and toes must therefore be checked regularly and carefully.

2. Regional analgesia is of value in the post-operative management of patients with chronic respiratory insufficiency due to myopathy, cystic fibrosis, Werdnig-Hoffmann disease or broncho-pulmonary dysplasia. In these and similar condi-tions, epidural analgesia facilitates chest physio-therapy and avoids the need for systemic opiates with their depressant effect on respiration (23).

3. Patients undergoing major abdominal and thoracic procedures, such as pull-through opera-tions, thoracotomies, Nissen procedures and resections of large tumours, require intensive nursing care, physiotherapy and other procedures. Epidural analgesia enables these to be carried out with minimal distress.

4. It has recently been shown that regional anae-thesia can be a valuable technique for the trauma-tised child. Fractures of the femoral shaft occur quite frequently in children and are very painful. In these cases, femoral nerve block appears to be effective and safe (26). The resulting analgesia, which was rated from 'good' to 'excellent' in the patients studied, allows positioning for X-ray examination, application of traction and general nursing care to be carried out painlessly.

Side-effects

Hypotension
Although this is very common in adults, it is unusual in children (24, 25).

Urinary retention
This also is unusual in children, but is more likely to occur if a continuous infusion is used instead of intermittent bolus top-ups.

Infection

A good sterile technique and an occlusive dressing for the catheter should ensure that this does not occur.

Systemic toxicity of the local anaesthetic
Knowledge of the pharmacokinetic properties of the drug and correct use of an appropriate technique are vital if this is to be avoided.

The side-effects of epidural opiates are considered later in this chapter.

Regional techniques for outpatient surgery

Methods
Regional anaesthesia has been widely used and extensively studied in children undergoing common, minor surgical procedures such as circumcision and inguinal hernia repair (5, 8, 11,12). For these cases, the most appropriate central block is the caudal, which can be per-formed either before or at the end of surgery. Of the peripheral blocks, penile and ilio-inguinal blocks are popular (27, 28, 29).

All these methods provide post-operative analgesia lasting 6 to 24 hours after a single injection

Table 15. Effects and side effects

Effects and side effects	Epidural opioids	Epidural local anaesthetics
Pain relief	Good Prolonged	Complete Less prolonged
Cardio-vascular	Minor changes Intact baroreflex response	minor changes in children under 8 for block up to T4. For children over 8 possible postural hypotension
Respira-tory	early depress (1-2h) (systemic absorpt) late depress (6-24h) (migration of opioids in CSF to brain).	no
CNS sedation other neuro-logical abnor malities	± to ++ Possible	no no
Convulsions	+ (very high dose)	Yes if rapid vascu-lar absorption
Various nausea vomiting urinary retention pruritis	+++ +++ +++ ± not usual in children	· + + + no

Adapted from Cousins and Mather Anesthesiology 1984; 61: 276-310

Fig. 119. The effects of age and addition of epinephrine to bupivacaine for caudal analgesia in pediatric patients. Warner (1985) Anesthesiology 63:A464

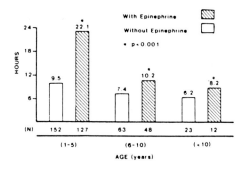

(8-12). Other peripheral blocks, such as brachial plexus, femoral and intercostal, have not been widely used in young children, but they are now increasing in popularity (30).

Drugs

Bupivacaine

Bupivacaine is the local anaesthetic drug of choice for post-operative analgesia because of its long duration of action and its sparing effect on motor fibres (31, 32). It is now universally agreed that caudal morphine should be avoided for paediatric outpatients because of the risk of delayed respiratory depression (10, 11).

Regional techniques after major surgery

Epidural anaesthesia is the most suitable and interesting technique for continuous use in children, and a considerable amount of informa-tion is now available about it (25). A catheter can be introduced into the lumbar and thoracic regions either before or after surgery and safely left there afterwards. Caudal catheters, if they are inserted at all, arc usually withdrawn at the end of the operation after a final top-up because their proximity to the anus renders them liable to infection.

Recently, the use of an intrapleural catheter for the relief of pain after upper abdominal and thoracic surgery has been reported. The catheter can be inserted by the surgeon during operation, or by the anaesthetist afterwards. The negative intrapleural pressure enables the space to be easily recognised by the loss of resistance test. A continuous infusion of 0.25% bupivacaine provides unilateral analgesia which facilitates postoperative care in these cases (33).

Post-operative analgesia can be provided by either epidural local anaesthetics or opiates and each has some advantages and disadvantages (34). These are summarised in Table 15.

Local anaesthetics

The two chief advantages of local anaesthetics are that they provide analgesia of excellent quality and they do not cause respiratory depression. There are several disadvantages. Repeated top-up injections are necessary at frequent intervals because even the longer acting agents may not last more than a few hours. If a continuous infusion is used to overcome this difficulty. undesirable motor block may occur even though dilute solutions are used. Tachyphylaxis is also a possibility.

Intermittent top-up injections are not recommended in adult patients (15) because, if tachyphylaxis occurs and increments need to be given more frequently and in larger dosage, there is a risk of systemic toxicity. There is also the risk of hypotension following top-ups which necessitates the maintenance of an intravenous infusion and, possibly, active treatment with a vasopressor. Finally, intermittent top-up injec-tions have to be very precisely timed if break-through pain is to be avoided.

Fortunately, these problems are not commonly seen in children. In the author's experience of more than 300 cases, neither tachyphylaxis nor hypotension have been observed (25). A continuous infusion can be administered by a syringe pump or a powered intravenous infusion pump. The latter is the more reliable because it is better able to overcome the resistance provided by the small gauge paediatric epidural catheter.

At the moment, very few studies of the effects of epidural infusions are available in children (35), so the safety of the technique is open to question. In particular, it has been noted that there is very wide variation in the amount of analgesia required even after major surgery, and many children do not seem to need further local anaesthetic in the first 24 hours post-operatively although, with an epidural catheter in place, it would be very easy to give it. There are two further risks. The child's dura is thinner and less resistant than that of the adult, so it is theoretically more likely to be punctured by the catheter during the course of an infusion. There is also the possibility that accumulation of infused bupivacaine may lead to very high plasma concentrations. This has been reported in an adult receiving 0.125% bupivacaine by infusion (36). Since no pharmacokinetic data are available for children, it is impossible to predict whether the

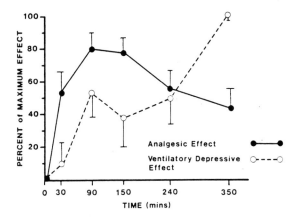

Fig. 120. Time courses of analgesic and ventilatory depressive effects of lumbar epidural morphine. Knill (1981) Can. Anaesth. Soc. J. 28:537

same thing would happen, so it is important to observe the child closely for signs of toxicity and, ideally, to monitor the plasma bupivacaine concentration. Clearly, further studies are required before this technique can be recommended whole-heartedly for children.

Bupivacaine is the drug of choice for post-operative analgesia by the epidural route. The concentration should not exceed 0.25% if motor block is to be avoided. No motor block has been observed in the author's cases when this concentration has been given by intermittent injection. The addition of adrenaline 1:200.000 prolongs the duration of the block (25, 32). In most children, the first top-up was needed at the 6th post-operative hour and the second between the 18th and 24th hour. The volume for top-up injections was half that used during surgery and it was found that this gave complete control of pain.

Etidocaine is a long-acting local anaesthetic, but it has two disadvantages. Firstly, its high lipid solubility results in profound motor block, and secondly, systemic toxicity may occur because repeated top-ups may lead to accumulation in the epidural space (37).

If the epidural catheter is inserted after the operation, the tip should be placed close to the nerves innervating the surgical field. This will ensure that analgesia is produced over the entire affected area with a comparatively small amount of local anaesthetic.

Opioids

The analgesic effect of epidural opioids was first reported by Yaksh and Rudy (38) in 1976. Since then, many other reports (most of them anecdotal) have appeared which document both their efficacy and their side-effects. Cousins and Mather (34) have recently reviewed the literature.

The advantages claimed for the opioids are that they provide longer post-operative analgesia than any long-acting local anaesthetic drug, and do not produce sympathetic or motor block. The most important disadvantage, especially in the case of morphine, is that they cause delayed respiratory depression due to rostral migration in the CSF (39, 40) (Fig. 120). This effect is antagonised by naloxone. When given in a dose of $10\mu g.kg^{-1}.h^{-1}$, naloxone prevents respiratory depression without reducing the analgesic effect in adults and children over 12 years of age (41, 42). There is unfortunately no information about younger patients, but if this technique is used in children, they must be carefully monitored in the post-operative period and close attention must be paid to respiratory rate and blood gases (43). As in adults, there are other undesirable side-effects such as nausea and vomiting, but pruritus is uncommon in children less than 8 years. The opioid can be given into the lumbar or thoracic region, but as the drug tends to spread rostrally, there is no advantage in using the thoracic route.

Preservative-free morphine, diluted in saline, is recommended for children over 6 years in a dose of $50~\mu g.kg^{-1}$. A single injection can be expected to last between 8 and 24 hours. No data regarding dosage are available for younger children, though the study by Shapiro (44) did include two children under 6 years. The present author has found that morphine in a dose of $25~\mu g.kg^{-1}$ provides good analgesia for 8 to 12 hours in children less than 3 years, but an increase in $PaCO_2$ and a decrease in respiratory rate were observed in most cases. It is therefore best to admit these children to an intensive care unit for the first 48 post-operative hours.

Fentanyl, unlike morphine, is highly lipid-soluble so the onset of analgesia is more rapid, and the duration of action shorter, than with morphine. Fentanyl $100\mu g$ provides analgesia for a mean of 3.83 hours in adults. The risk of respiratory depression is theoretically smaller with a lipid-soluble drug.

Summary

1. Local anaesthetics provide complete and prolonged pain control, and when 0.25% bupivacaine is used, side effects are minimal. Comprehensive pharmacokinetic data are available for caudals and epidurals in children.

2. Epidural morphine is an acceptable alternative in children over 10 years provided that they are carefully monitored. It is valuable for pain relief after traumatic injuries.

3. The other opioids do not seem to offer any particular advantage over morphine in adults, but further information is needed before any definite conclusions can be drawn (45, 46).

References

1. Abu-Saad H (1984) Assessing children's responses to pain. Pain 19:163

2. Owens ME (1984) Pain in infancy:conceptual and methodological issues. Pain 20:213

3. Mather L, Mackie J (1983) The incidence of postoperative pain in children. Pain 15:271

4. Booker PD, Nightingale DA (1985) Post-operative analgesia in children in: The management of postoperative pain. Edited by ME Dobson, Edwards Arnold Publishers p 200

5. Kay B (1974) Caudal block for postoperative pain relief in children. Anaesthesia 29:610

6. Shandling B, Steward DJ (1980) Regional analgesia for postoperative pain in pediatric outpatient surgery. J Pediatr Surg 15:477

7. Anderson R (1976) Pain as a major cause of post-operative nausea. Canad Anaesth Soc J 23:366

8. Hannalah RS, Broadman LM, Belman AB, Abramowitz MD, Epstein BS (1987) Comparison of caudal and ilioinguinal/iliohypogastric nerve blocks for control of post-orchidopexy pain in pediatric ambulatory surgery. Anesthesiology 66.832

9. Yeoman PM, Cooke R, Hain WR (1983) Penile block for circumcision ? A comparison with caudal blockade. Anaesthesia 38:862

10. Tree-Trakarn, T Pirayavaraporn S (1985) Post-operative pain relief for circumcision in children: comparison among morphine nerve block and topical analgesia. Anesthesiology 62:519

11. Jensen BH (1981) Caudal block for post-operative pain relief in children after genital operations. A comparison between bupivacaine and morphine. Acta Anaesth Scand 25:373

12. Fell D, Derrington MC, Taylor E, Wandless JG (1988) Paediatric postoperative analgesia. A comparison between caudal block and wound infiltration of local anaesthetic. Anaesthesia 43:107

13. Armitage EN (1985) Regional anaesthesia. Clin Anesthesiol 3:553

14. Schulte Steinberg O (1980) Neural blockade for pediatric surgery in: Neural blockade in clinical anesthesia and Pain management. Eds Cousins MJ, Bridenbaugh PO. Lippincott, Philadelphia, Chapter 21, p 503

15. Pither C, Hartrick C (1985) Post-operative pain. In: Handbook of regional anesthesia, p 99. Edited by PP Raj. Churchill-Livingstone Publishers

16. Kehlet H (1984) The stress response to anaesthesia and surgery: Release mechanisms and modifying factors. Clinics in Anaesthesiology 2:315

17. Asoh T, Tsuji H, Shirasaka C, Takenchi Y (1983) Effect of epidural analgesia on metabolic response to major upper abdominal surgery. Acta Anaesth Scand 27:233

18. Murat I, Walker J, Esteve C, Nahoul K, Saint-Maurice C (1988) Effect of lumbar epidural anaesthesia on plasma cortisol levels in children. Can Anaesth Soc J 35:20

19. Koren G, Butt W, Chinyanga H, Soldin S, Tan YK, Pape K (1985) Postoperative morphine infusion in newborn infants: Assessment of disposition characteristics and safety. J Pediatr 107:963

20. Benhamou D, Samii K, Noviant Y (1983) Effect of analgesia on respiratory muscle function after upper abdominal surgery. Acta Anaesth Scand 27:22

21. Simpson BR, Parkhouse J, Marshall R, Lambrechts W (1961) Extradural analgesia and the prevention of post-operative pain. Br J Anaesth 33:628

22. Pflug AE, Murphy TM, Butler SH, Tucker GT (1974) The effects of post-operative peridural analgesia in pulmonary therapy and pulmonary complications. Anesthesiology 41:20

23. Meignier M, Souron R, Le Neel JC (1983) Post-operative dorsal epidural analgesia in the child with respiratory disabilities. Anesthesiology 59:473

24. Arthur DS (1980) Post-operative thoracic epidural analgesia in children. Anaesthesia 35:1131

25. Murat I, Delleur MM, Esteve C, Egu JF, Raynaud P, Saint-Maurice C (1987) Continuous extradural anaesthesia in children. Br J Anaesth 59:1441

26. Ronchi L, Rosenbaum D, Lenormand Y, Lemaitre JL, Guillet JC (1986) Femoral nerve block with bupivacaine in children. Anesthesiology 65:A430

27. Hinkle AJ (1987) Percutaneous inguinal block

for the outpatient management of post-herniorrhaphy pain in children. Anesthesiology 67:411

28. Carlsson P, Svensson J (1984) The duration of pain relief after penile block to boys undergoing circumcision. Acta Anaesth Scand 28:432

29. Soliman MG, Tremblay NA (1978) Nerve block of the penis for post-operative pain relief in children. Anesth Analg 57:495

30. McNicol LR (1985) Sciatic nerve block for children. Sciatic nerve block by the anterior approach for postoperative pain relief. Anaesthesia 40:410

31. Wolf AR, Valley RD, Fear DW, Roy WL, Lerman J (1988) Bupivacaine for caudal analgesia in infants and children: the optimal effective concentration. Anesthesiology 69:102

32. Warner MA, Kunkel SE, Offord KO, Atchinson SR, Dawson B (1987) The effects of age, epinephrine, and operative site on duration of caudal analgesia in pediatric patients. Anesth Analg 66:995

33. McIlvaine WB, Knox RF, Fennessey PV, Goldstein M (1988) Continuous infusion of bupivacaine via intrapleural catheter for analgesia after thoracotomy in children. Anesthesiology 69:261

34. Cousins MJ, Mather LE (1984) Intrathecal and epidural administration of opioids. Anesthesiology 61:276

35. Desparmet J, Meistelman C, Barre J, Saint-Maurice C (1987) Continuous epidural infusion of bupivacaine for postoperative pain relief in children. Anesthesiology 67:108

36. Richter O, Klein K, Abel J, Ohnesorge FK, Wust HJ, Thiessen FMM (1984) The kinetics of bupivacaine plasma concentrations during epidural anesthesia following intra-operative bolus injection and subsequent continuous infusion. Int J Clin Pharmacol Ther 22:611

37. Tucker GT, Cooper S, Littlewood D, Buckley FP, Covino BG (1977) Observed and predicted accumulation of local anaesthetic during continuous extradural analgesia. Br J Anaesth 49:237

38. Yaksh TL, Rudy TA (1976) Analgesia mediated by a direct spinal action of narcotics. Science 192:1357

39. Catley DM, Thornton C, Tech JB, Lehane JR, Royston D, Jones JG (1985) Pronounced episodic oxygen desaturation in the postoperative period: its association with ventilatory pattern and analgesic regimen. Anesthesiology 63:20

40. Knill RL, Clement Vl, Thompson WR (1981) Epidural morphine causes delayed and prolonged respiratory depression. Canad Anaesth Soc J 28:537

41. Finholt DA, Stirt JA, DiFazio CA (1985) Epidural morphine for postoperative analgesia in pediatric patients. Anesth Analg 64:211

42. Rawal N, Schott U, Dahlström B, Inturrisi CE, Tandon B, Sjöstrand U, Wennhager M (1986) Influence of naloxone infusion on analgesia and respiratory depression following epidural morphine. Anesthesiology 64:194

43. Attia J, Ecoffey C, Sandouk P, Gross JB, Samii K (1986) Epidural morphine in children: pharmacokinetics and CO_2 sensitivity. Anesthesiology 65:590

44. Shapiro LA, Jedeikin RJ, Shalev D, Hoffmaan S (1984) Epidural morphine analgesia in children. Anesthesiology 61:210

45. Benlabed M, Ecoffey C, Levron JC, Flaisler B, Gross JB (1987) Analgesia and ventilatory response to CO_2 following epidural sufentanil in children. Anesthesiology 67:948

46. Whiting WC, Sandler AN, Lau LC, Chovaz PM, Slavchenko P, Daley D, Koren G (1988) Analgesic and respiratory effects of epidural sufentanil in patients following thoracotomy. Anesthesiology 69:36

Chronic pain

Michel Meignier and

Ottheinz Schulte Steinberg

Although chronic pain is a well known clinical entity in adults, it is largely unrecognised in children and very little information is available about it. Similarly, the use of local anaesthetic techniques in the treatment of chronic pain in children is recent and the subject is poorly documented. Most of our experience of local anaesthetics in children has been obtained during operative surgery and in the immediate post-operative period.

"Pain is an uncomfortable sensorial and emotional experience associated with real or apparent tissue damage or described in terms of such damage" (1). Children up to the age of 15 years presenting with chronic pain are almost always suffering from an invasive, neoplastic process. It is very rare for there to be any other cause.

The pain may appear at any stage in the illness. It may be the first presenting symptom or it may herald recurrence of the condition after initial treatment and, of course, it may be a feature of the terminal phase.

Pain arises principally from compression or invasion of nerves, bones and viscera. It may also arise from raised intracranial pressure due to intracranial tumours. Chronic pain, which may last for weeks or months, considerably affects the whole attitude of the child to his illness, and this makes the condition very difficult to treat.

Pain is the result of an imbalance between excitatory and inhibitory stimulation. Nociceptive information from mechanical or chemical stimuli is transmitted along the nerve by small diameter A and C fibres. Neurochemical inhibition of these stimuli may be mediated peripherally by prostaglandin F and centrally by endorphins. Neurophysiological inhibition is exerted by the opposing effects of discharge from the large diameter fibres and the small diameter A and C fibres. These mechanisms are important for the understanding of the effects of local anaesthetics in the relief of pain.

It will be seen from the above that there are two types of pain. One type results from the prolonged stimulation of nociceptors. Clinically, it is acute and well localised, and the patient's response is usually proportional to its severity. The other type results from absence of inhibition due to transection of inhibitory pathways or to demyelination of large fibres. Clinically, it presents as a burning sensation or causalgia, and the patient may show abnormal psychological responses to it. Both types of pain may appear, together or separately, during the course of malignant disease, and both of them are amenable to treatment by regional analgesic techniques.

In children, the incidence of chronic pain is rare compared with adults, but even if we believe that a child suffers less pain after straight-forward surgery, there is no reason to believe it suffers less when the pain is due, say, to an osteosarcoma or to the intra-abdominal spread of a neuroblastoma.

Chronic pain in infants is not well treated because it is not a well recognised clinical condition. Unlike the child in acute pain, the child suffering from chronic pain will never talk about it and may even deny that he has it. He becomes introverted and very often tries to erect barriers between himself and the medical team. However, close observation of these infants shows them to be apathetic and withdrawn. It seems that, in order to tolerate his suffering, the child has to detach and isolate himself and become cocooned off from his surroundings so that he assumes an almost comatose attitude. If treatment is to be effective therefore, the physician must first be aware that the condition exists before he can identify it in his patients. Once the diagnosis has been made, the support of several different specialists - psychologists, paediatric psychiatrists and all the members of the medical team - is necessary. Regional analgesia can play an important part within the overall treatment plan.

Regional techniques for chronic pain

All the methods used must have as their objective the interruption of pain conduction pathways. As a first step, transcutaneous nerve stimulation may be tried. If this is unsuccessful, the pathways can be interrupted by nerve block which can be achieved either by the use of a catheter to provide continuous analgesia with reversible agents such as local anaesthetics and narcotics, or by the use of a neurolytic agent to destroy the somatic or sympathetic pathways. In the first case, the duration of analgesia in the short term will depend on the pharmacology of the drug, but in the long term the main limiting factor is the life of the catheter. In the second case, the effect of the chemical neurolysis lasts very considerably longer, but unfortunately the anaesthetist has less control over the final result.

Regional blocks with a catheter

Epidural analgesia

Analgesia may be administered by the lumbar or thoracic route. Access to the epidural space presents no special difficulties and the technique is the same as that used for operative surgery and for postoperative analgesia. The caudal route is unsuitable because a catheter remaining in place for several days is in danger of becoming infected due to the proximity of the anus.

At first sight, it might seem that, if a catheter is to remain in place for a very long time, polyurethane or silicone would be the materials of choice. In fact, experience obtained with adults (and confirmed in children) suggests that the type of material is not so important and nylon has also been found to be satisfactory. The size of the catheter should be appropriate to the child.

If the catheter is likely to be in place for more than a week, it is advisable to tunnel it subcutaneously so that it emerges from the skin at some distance from its entry point and at a site where it is unlikely to be disturbed by excessive movement. It should be firmly fixed to avoid any damage. A light, occlusive hypo-allergenic dressing should be applied. Experience with long-term intravenous catheters suggests that dressings should be replaced every three days unless there are clinical reasons for it more frequently.

A modification of the epidural catheter technique is the use of narcotic sachets implanted subcutaneously. The sachets are connected to the epidural catheter and, when empty, they can be refilled by direct injection through the skin with a subcutaneous needle. The advantage is that the sachet and catheter form a closed system so the risk of infection is reduced. However, with the possible exception of adolescents, the method is not particularly suitable for children, because the refilling of the sachet, involving another injection, is an extra source of anxiety and pain.

Epidural analgesia is most effective for pain in the abdomen, pelvis and lower limb, but it is less suitable for pain in the foot. The choice of drug lies between local anaesthetics and narcotics, and the phase and severity of the illness will dictate which agent is used. In the early phase of chronic pain, for example after surgery, local anaesthetics are preferred (0.25% bupivacaine with or without adrenaline in a dose of 4-6mg.kg^{-1} day^{-1}) (2,3), because they are well tolerated and it is easy to adjust the dose. On the other hand, during the terminal phase of the illness, narcotics are more appropriate (morphine 50-100µg.kg^{-1} day^{-1}) (4,5,6) as they avoid the need for other analgesics. They can either be administered intermittently, at a pre-determined time or when required, or continuously by an infusion pump. For chronic pain, the latter method is preferable and portable pumps are particularly useful because, being small, they allow the child to be fully mobile and even to return home.

Spinal analgesia

The lumbar or thoracic intrathecal approach has no place in the management of chronic pain in children. Although it is not difficult to perform, it offers no advantages over epidural analgesia yet it may give rise to complications of its own, such as loss of CSF and intrathecal compressive haematoma. Similarly, intraventricular catheters have very little place in paediatric practice. They may be indicated in the treatment of resistant head and neck pain, but this is fortunately rare in children except in cases of neuroblastoma and head and neck sarcoma. An additional disadvantage is that a separate surgical procedure is required for the insertion of the catheter

Continuous brachial plexus block

This technique is very suitable for the analgesic management of large tumours of the arm and serious joint pains. The axillary approach is used and is quite simple to perform (7). A catheter is passed into the axillary sheath where it can safely be maintained because the absence of hair and sweating in the child's axilla reduces the risk of infection.

There is, however, the possibility that the catheter will become displaced and, in practice, this usually limits the duration of the technique to 6 to 10 days. Children receiving continuous axillary block tend to become very dependent on it and are reluctant to make any movements (8). Plain bupivacaine 0.25% is given in a dose of 0.5-1ml.kg^{-1}.day^{-1}.

Intercostal nerve blocks

These are of use in the analgesic management of soft tissue tumours which have invaded the parietal tissues. The posterior approach is best because it enables the lateral cutaneous branch to be blocked. The introduction of a catheter into the intercostal groove has been described (9) and continuous analgesia can be obtained by perfusing 0.25% bupivacaine in a dose of 0.2-0.5ml.kg^{-1}.day^{-1}. As with brachial plexus block, the catheter may become displaced and this limits the usefulness of the technique.

Tibial and perineal nerve blocks

Block of these nerves in the popliteal fossa is useful for manipulation of the feet in spastic patients and it has been shown that earlier walking can be achieved when this technique is used (10).

Regional blocks with chemical agents

Somatic blocks

Partial or total neurolysis of somatic nerves is indicated when pain results from excessive nociception due to involvement of a nerve in the strictly local spread of a malignant tumour. They are long-lasting and are therefore very suitable for children with chronic pain who have a reasonably long life expectancy.

There are, however, many important disadvantages. It is very difficult to predict how effective (extensive) the block will be, or whether sensory or motor fibres will be the most affected. Since motor block may be produced, the technique is best reserved for children who already have some motor deficit. Another unfortunate feature is that neuritic pains may appear several weeks or months after the block, and these are very difficult to treat. Neurolytic axillary and intercostal blocks may be performed, using the standard techniques, with 5 or 10% aqueous phenol or absolute alcohol (10).

Sympathetic blocks

These are useful for pain arising from the thoracic and upper abdominal viscera. As the nociceptive impulses are partly transmitted along efferent sympathetic fibres, destruction of these fibres interrupts pain conduction.

Coelio-splanchnic block

This is indicated where there is direct compression of the ganglia by the tumour, and where the tumour has invaded organs (such as the pancreas, stomach and liver) which the ganglia subserve. It is a dangerous technique and should only be performed under X-ray control. The child lies prone with a pillow under the abdomen. A 20G spinal needle is introduced from a lateral position and is directed anteriorly and medially. 1-2ml of 1% lidocaine is injected first because this renders the subsequent injection of 0.25 - 0.35ml.kg^{-1} of absolute alcohol less painful (11).

The aorta is closely related to the coeliac plexus. It is therefore wise to verify the position of the needle radiographically by the prior injection of contrast medium, and to aspirate repeatedly during the injection of the alcohol. Since there is a risk of tissue necrosis along the track of the needle, it must be syringed through with saline before it is withdrawn.

Pain relief occurs 24 to 36 hours after the injection. Side effects during this period are very important and include hypotension, bowel distension and vomiting. The use of vasopressors for treatment of the hypotension is dangerous, but an abdominal binder is sometimes helpful.

Stellate Ganglion Block
This is indicated for pain arising from oedema associated with malignant invasion in the lower part of the neck, the mediastinum and the lung.
The ganglion is approached at the level of the seventh cervical vertebra and 2 to 5ml of absolute alcohol are injected. Stellate ganglion block has also been successfully used to treat arterial insufficiency in the arm of a two week old premature infant. One injection of local anaesthetic was sufficient in this case (12).

Intravenous regional anaesthesia
Guanethidine may be given by this route for the treatment of reflex sympathetic dystrophy. For example, a girl of 8 years received guanethidine 10mg in saline 20ml (13). However, the result was not long-lasting, and sympathetic blocks were eventually needed.

Lumbar sympathetic block
In the case just described, the lumbar sympathetic chain was blocked at L2-4 with 0.5% bupivacaine followed at a later date by 4ml of phenol 10%. It is of course essential that the correct position of the needles is confirmed radiologically. In addition to the typical features of the disease, demineralisation of the bones and retardation of bone growth were observed by the authors at the commencement of treatment. During the year following treatment, recovery of growth was seen (13).

Drug metabolism in the severely ill child
No information is available regarding the pharmacokinetics of local anaesthetic or narcotic drugs in children with major metabolic disturbances. However, it seems logical to suggest the use of reduced doses in cases of severe protein deficiency. When the dosage of a narcotic is being considered, liver function should be taken into account, as should the concurrent administration of certain antibiotics and cyclosporine.

Place of regional anaesthesia
Regional analgesia should not be used alone as the sole method of analgesia, nor should it be used in all cases of chronic pain. There are two typical situations in which it is of value.
Firstly, it can be used to overcome a particularly painful period, for example, immediately after surgery. Where possible, a technique should be used which allows the use of a catheter. The results are so successful that this is the method of choice and it should be tried first. Secondly, regional analgesia may be included in the treatment of pain against the background of chronic illness, and in these circumstances it will be integrated with other analgesics in the overall treatment plan. Oral narcotics, given by mouth, can provide excellent analgesia. They are very well tolerated and there is no risk of dependance. If very large doses are required, a continuous block should be considered as this may enable the dose to be reduced and may avoid the need for intravenous narcotic administration and its attendant undesirable side-effects. Sympathetic and neurolytic blocks are useful in special circumstances.

Hence, when the indications are being considered, a clear distinction should be made between the management of the acute phase and the terminal phase of a child's pain, although in both instances the anaesthetist's aim is to relieve the child. Similarly, the contraindications should be assessed in relation to the child's life expectancy. In the early, acute phase, conditions such as a low platelet count or imperfect skin at the site of needle insertion would be valid contraindications, but in the terminal phase, a child should be given the benefit of regional analgesia inspite of these contraindications, so that he can die in comfort and with dignity.

Conclusion

Chronic pain in children is almost certainly underestimated because it is not well recognised.

Experience gained with regional anaesthetic techniques during and immediately after surgery have allowed their development for the management of chronic pain.

The choice of technique, the precise time at which it is introduced, and the drug used should all take into account the state of the child and his life expectancy.

Regional techniques should be integrated into a very well defined scheme for pain control which should include the constant psychological support of the child and his family. They can help in avoiding the child being subjected to "another invasive procedure".

Pain is a very common symptom, but under these circumstances it fulfils no biological function and conveys no benefit to the child. It follows therefore that it should always be treated.

References

1. Merskey H (1979) Pain terms: a list with definitions and note on usage. Pain 6: 249
2. Desparmet J, Meistelman C, Barre J, Saint-Maurice C (1986) Continuous epidural infusion of bupivacaine for post- operative pain relief in children. Anesthesiology 65:3A:424
3. Meigner M, Souron R, Le Neel JC (1983) Post-operative dorsal epidural analgesia in the child with respiratory disabilities. Anesthesiology 55:473
4. Glenski JA, Warner MA, Dawson B, Kaufman B (1984) Postoperative use of epidurally administered morphine in children and adolescents. Mayo Clinic Proc 59:530
5. Ecoffey C, Attia J, Samii K (1985) Analgesia and side effects following epidural morphine in children Anesthesiology 63:470
6. Shapiro LA, Jedeikin RJ, Shaley (1984) Epidural morphine in children. Anesthesiology 61:210
7. Selander D (1977) Catheter technique in axillary plexus block. Acta Anaesth Scand 21:324
8. Rosenblatt R, Pepitone-Rockwell F, McKillop MJ (1979) Continuous axillary analgesia for traumatic hand injury. Anesthesiology 51:565
9. Moore DC (1981) Intercostal nerve block: spread of india ink injected to the rib costal groove. Brit J Anaesth 53:325
10. Kempthorne PM, Brown TCK (1984) Nerve blocks around the knee in children. Anaesth Intens Care 12:14
11. Moore DC (1975) Regional block. Fourth edition. C.C. Thomas ed, Springfield Illinois.
12. Lagade MRG, Poppers PJ (1984) Stellate ganglion block: a therapeutic modality for arterial insufficiency of the arm in premature infants. Anesthesiology 61:203
13. Doolan LA, Brown TCK (1984) Reflex sympathetic dystrophy in a child. Anaesth Intens Care 12:70

IV Uncommon diseases & special problems

Respiratory tract

Isabelle Murat

Conditions affecting airway management

Elective and emergency surgical procedures have sometimes to be carried out in children who have compromised airways. The potential difficulties can usually be recognised before anaesthesia, and they include obstructive masses, macroglossia, micrognathia, limited mobility of the mouth and jaw, and symptoms such as stridor (Table 16). The nature and severity of the pathology must be carefully assessed at the pre-operative visit.

The place of regional anaesthesia in the management of these conditions depends on the proposed surgical procedure, the age of the child, and the likely complications of both regional and general anaesthesia - if regional and general anaesthesia are to be combined, it is essential that the airway is entrusted to a competent assistant while the block is being performed. However, some guidelines can be drawn up.

Minor procedures

For minor procedures on the perineum and lower limbs, a single-shot caudal injection is the technique of choice in young children of less than 30kg. The injection itself is easy and the incidence of failure and complications is very low. Small babies can be firmly held while the block is being performed. Older children require sedation and, in some cases, infiltration of local anaesthetic down to the sacro-coccygeal membrane.

Major procedures

For major procedures, intubation may be essential and it may have to be performed under topical anaesthesia or with a fibre-optic device, and general anaesthesia is not administered until the airway has been safely secured. Even in these cases, regional anaesthesia does have a valuable role because it enables the general anaesthesia to be maintained with reduced amounts of muscle relaxant and opiate drugs. The result is that the child awakes promptly and with full muscle tone, so the risk of upper airway obstruction and respiratory depression in the immediate postoperative period is minimised.

Table 16. Congenital causes of upper airway obstruction in children

---

Choanal atresia
Cranio-facial malformations
      Pierre Robin syndrome
      Treacher Collins syndrome
      Goldenhar syndrome
Macroglossia
      Down's syndrome
      Beckwith's syndrome
      mucopolysaccharidoses
Laryngeal
      laryngomalacia
      subglottic stenosis
      laryngo-tracheo-oesophageal cleft
      cord palsies
Tracheal
      tracheomalacia
      congenital stenosis
Congenital tumours and cysts
      haemangioma
      lymphangioma
      cystic hygroma

Intermediate procedures

For intermediate procedures, the choice of technique will be influenced by the intelligence and age of the child, on the surgical procedure to be performed and on the training of the paediatric anaesthesia staff.

All cases

For all cases, the anaesthetist must ensure that it is possible to maintain the airway using a facemask before carrying out regional anaesthesia.

Conditions causing respiratory insufficiency

Respiratory insufficiency can give rise to problems both during and after operation. It may be caused by intrinsic lung disease, by muscle weakness or by chest wall deformities. Most of these conditions are described in the chapter on the myopathies (p. 190). The general principles of their management are the same as for the management of the difficult airway.

Special care is necessary for premature infants who sometimes need surgery for hernia repair, often under emergency conditions. These infants are more prone to complications after general anaesthesia than full term babies (1) and apnoea may occur even after minor surgery (2). In such cases, caudal anaesthesia under light sedation is appropriate since it avoids the need for tracheal intubation and is easy to perform in this age group.

Spinal anaesthesia has been recommended (3,4) for the high risk neonate, but there is as yet little information on the haemodynamic and respiratory consequences of this technique. No obvious advantage over the caudal is apparent (5), though the dose of drug required for a spinal is much less.

References

1. Steward DJ (1982) Preterm infants are more prone to complications following minor surgery than term infants. Anesthesiology 56:304
2. Liu Lmp, Cote JC, Goudsouzian NG, Ryan JF, Firestone S, Debrick DF, Liu PL, Todres D (1983) Life threatening apnea in infants recovering from anesthesia. Anesthesiology 59:506
3. Abajian JC, Mellish I, Browne AE, Perkins FM, Lamberg DH, Mazuzan JE (1984) Spinal anesthesia for the high risk infant Anesth Analg 63:359
4. Blaise G, Roy L (1985) Spinal anesthesia in pediatric surgery. Anesth Analg 64:196
5. Mayhew JF, Moreno L (1984) Spinal anesthesia for high risk neonate. Letter to the editor of Anesth Analg 63:782

Neurological conditions

Ottheinz Schulte Steinberg

General considerations

Before individual diseases are considered, some important general points need to be mentioned. Neurological sequelae attributable to regional blocks invariably attract widespread publicity.

The vast majority of these mishaps are due to a fault in the drugs or equipment used or to some aspect of the management of the case. The incidence of life-threatening complications after regional anaesthesia is very low indeed, and is only about one third of those occurring during general anaesthesia. Nevertheless, the prospect of adverse publicity and possible litigation naturally makes anaesthetists reluctant to use regional anaesthesia in patients with pre-existing neurological pathology.

Care must obviously be taken to avoid complications arising from the mechanical effects of injections, such as the dangerous increase in intracranial pressure which may occur with subarachnoid injections in cases of brain tumour, but these precautions apply to all solutions and not specifically to local anaesthetics. It must therefore be stressed that local anaesthetic solutions have been shown not to cause any nerve damage or tissue change, provided that they are uncontaminated and given in the recommended clinical concentrations. It follows that these solutions, deposited distant from the site of the neurological pathology, will not adversely affect the course of the underlying condition.

When regional anaesthesia is being considered in a child with neurological disease, it is essential to have an explicit and honest discussion of the situation with the parents. The risks and potential advantages of the technique have to be explained to them, and these have then to be weighed against a general anaesthetic. Prior to regional anaesthesia, a full expert neurological examination is mandatory. This is the only way of establishing the preoperative extent of the deficit - information which is essential in the unfortunate event of litigation at a later stage. Fear of possible litigation should not, however, influence the anaesthetist in his choice of anaesthetic technique and if, after full assessment, he feels that regional anaesthesia is best for the child, he should proceed.

Epilepsy

Although the cause of idiopathic epilepsy remains unknown, acquired epilepsy has an intracranial cause. There is therefore no reason to limit the use of regional anaesthesia except where the epilepsy is due to a brain tumour. Epileptic patients should be well sedated so that convulsions, which may mistakenly be attributed to the local anaesthetic, do not occur.

Genetic developmental and degenerative diseases

Cerebral palsy

This is no contraindication to the use of regional anaesthesia, provided that there is no clinical evidence of progressive deterioration of neurological function.

Friedreich's ataxia

In this condition, the degenerative process involves the spinal cord, and while no adverse effects of spinal or epidural anaesthesia should logically be expected, these techniques are best avoided, if only for medicolegal reasons.

Motor neurone diseases

Amyotrophic lateral sclerosis, progressive muscular atrophy, progressive bulbar palsy, primary lateral sclerosis as well as hereditary familial juvenile muscular atrophy and familial spastic paraplegia all involve degeneration of the structures of the cord. Despite lack of any evidence that central blocks are unsafe, they are again best avoided for medicolegal reasons.

Extrapyramidal disorders

Acute inflammatory chorea (Sydenham's or rheumatic fever chorea) and the chronic hereditary form (Huntington's) involve changes in the cerebral cortex and basal ganglia. Since the pathology is entirely intracranial, all forms of regional anaesthesia may be considered

Cerebrovascular diseases
The only example of this group likely to be found in children is subarachnoid haemorrhage. Regional anaesthesia is not necessarily contra-indicated provided that the blood pressure is kept stable, and this is not usually difficult in children, even with central blocks. Crawford (3,4) recommends the caudal approach in these cases because dural tap is less likely than with the higher epidural approach. Spinal anaesthesia seems inadvisable, but there is no contra-indication to peripheral blocks.

Infections and inflammatory diseases of CNS and meninges
These include meningitis, cerebral abscess, sub-dural empyema, cerebral epidural abscess, sinus thrombosis, spinal epidural infections, encepha-lomyelitis and syphilis. Spinal anaesthesia should be avoided. Where the infection is strictly limited to intracranial structures, other regional techniques may be used, but infection within the spinal canal precludes central blocks of any kind. Peripheral nerve blocks may be used.

Demyelinating diseases
Multiple sclerosis is the most important disease in this group and it can occur as early as the tenth year of life. The lesions are scattered throughout the brain and spinal cord. There is increasing evidence that epidural anaesthesia is quite well tolerated in these patients (1,2,4,5,6). It is also beneficial in clinical practice because the use of opioids and neuromuscular blocking agents can be reduced and, sometimes, avoided altogether. No information is available regarding peripheral blocks, but since the pathological lesions are remote from peripheral nerves, they may be expected to be harmless.

Intracranial tumours and raised intracranial pressure
Spinal and epidural anaesthesia should be avoided because of the danger that they might raise intracranial pressure and cause serious clinical deterioration. Regional anaesthesia should be limited to the use of peripheral nerve blocks.

Diseases of the spinal cord
Spinal and epidural anaesthesia are contra-indicated in the presence of active disease of the spinal cord. Epidural anaesthesia has been used without complications in cases such as residual poliomyelitis in which the active process has ceased (4). Peripheral blocks do not appear con-traindicated.

Diseases affecting spinal nerve roots
Chronic adhesive arachnoiditis is an absolute contraindication to central blocks. Mechanical compression of spinal nerve roots, on the other hand, is not necessarily a contraindication - indeed, in adults, laminectomy for the surgical treatment of herniated intervertebral discs is performed under epidural anaesthesia in some centres.

Diseases of peripheral nerves
Peripheral nerve neuropathies such as trigeminal neuralgia, sciatica and neuralgia paraesthetica benefit from peripheral blocks, but regional anaesthesia is not advisable in acute idiopathic polyneuropathy (also known as polyneuritis and Guillan-Barre Syndrome). However, Crawford administered epidural anaesthesia to two patients in the recovery phase of the disease and he encountered no complications (4).

Neuromuscular disorders

Myasthenia gravis
This presents the anaesthetist with considerable problems with regard to the use of muscle relaxants because the abnormality is at the neuro-muscular junction. Regional anaesthesia, both central and peripheral, may eliminate the need for muscle relaxants altogether and if an endotracheal tube is required, it can easily be passed under topical anaesthesia.

Dystrophia myotonica
Inability to relax muscle groups is believed to be due to an increased sensitivity of the muscle fibre (7). Both neostigmine and depolarising muscle relaxants may increase the degree of myotonia, while non-depolarising agents block neuro-muscular transmission without necessarily overcoming the myotonia. Furthermore, since

the defect is in the muscle itself, spinal and epidural block are also ineffective in overcoming the myotonia. However, peripheral nerve blocks are well tolerated.

Malignant hyperpyrexia

This is usually associated with clinical or subclinical myopathy, triggered by inhalation anaesthetics and muscle relaxants. Regional anaesthesia, with procaine or chloroprocaine, may enable the anaesthetist to avoid the use of these trigger agents, and such cases have been reported by Crawford (5), Khalil (8) and Willatts (9). It seems that lidocaine and other amide local anaesthetics can also be used safely (10). It is of paramount importance that all the spinal sympathetic outflow is blocked. An epidural catheter should therefore be inserted so that a block to the level of T1 may be obtained, and maintained for several hours postoperatively. Unless these precautions are taken, full protection is not achieved (9).

Familial Periodic Paralysis

This condition presents with weakness or paralysis of the limbs and is associated with potassium disturbances which may take a hypo- or hyper-kalaemic form. Attacks may be precipitated by succinylcholine in the hyperkalaemic type and by the administration of glucose, insulin and adrenaline in the hypokalaemic type. Regional anaesthesia is suitable for these patients.

Dermatomyositis

This condition results in profound peripheral muscle weakness, and Churchill-Davidson and colleagues (7) found evidence of a myasthenic response in some patients. Muscle relaxants should therefore be used with caution, and regional techniques are indicated.

Myositis OssificansProgressiva

The bony infiltration of tendons, aponeuroses and muscles can lead to ankylosis of the neck and cause difficulties with intubation. Regional anaesthesia may avoid the need for intubation.

References

1. Baskett PJF, Armstrong R (1970) Anaesthetic problems in multiple sclerosis. Are certain agents contraindicated. Anaesthesia 25:397
2. Frost PM (1971) Anaesthesia and Multiple Sclerosis (letter) Anaesthesia 26:104
3. Crawford JS (1978) Principles and Practice of Obstetric Anaesthesia p 365 4th ed. Blackwell
4. Crawford JS (1981) Regional analgesia for patients with chronic neurological disease and similar conditions. Anaesthesia 36:821
5. Crawford JS (1983) Epidural analgesia for patients with chronic neurological disease. Anesth Analg 62:617
6. Warren TM, Datta S and Ostheimer GW (1982) Lumbar epidural anaesthesia in a patient with multiple sclerosis. Anesth Analg 61:1022
7. Wylie WD and Churchill-Davidson HC (1972) A Practice of Anaesthesia. p 924 3rd ed. Lloyd-Luke (Medical Books) Ltd. London
8. Khalil SN, Williams JP and Bourke DL (1983) Management of a malignant hyperthermia susceptible patient in labor with 2- chloroprocaine epidural anesthesia. Anesth. Analg 62:115
9. Willatts SM (1979) Malignant hyperthermia susceptibility. Management during pregnancy and labour. Anaesthesia 34:41
10. Paasuke RT, Brownell AKW (1986) Amide local anaesthetics and malignant hyperthermia (editorial). Can Anaesth Soc J 33 (2):126
11. Bromage PR (1978) Epidural Analgesia. p 399. WB Saunders Company, Philadelphia, London

Allergy

Jean-Luc Hody

Introduction

Hypersensitivity, or true allergy, to local anaesthetics in children has yet to be described in the literature. Although there is no doubt that hypersensitivity can occur in adults in response to ester derivatives, it has been described, with supporting laboratory evidence, only once for amide local anaesthetics (1). On the other hand, adverse systemic reactions, mistakenly thought to be due to allergy, have been very fully documented. A patient with such symptoms is at risk of being labelled 'allergic' unless a careful history is taken and the correct diagnosis is established. Regional anaesthesia is too valuable to be denied to children simply on the basis of a history of allergy (2,3,4,5).

Adverse reactions to local anaesthetics

Adverse reactions to local anaesthetics may be defined as follows according to the response to the allergen:(Fig. 122)(6). It is not easy to diagnose an anaphylactic response to local anaesthetics (7,8) because it is sometimes difficult to distinguish the episode from cardio-vascular collapse due to toxicity induced by accidental intravenous injection, too high a dose or too rapid absorption. Early signs of toxicity, such as buccal, auditory and ocular symptoms, are often wrongly attributed to allergy by the patient.

Adrenaline

Adrenaline is frequently added to local anaesthetics and may cause an increase in plasma catecholamine levels. Alpha- and beta-adrenergic effects manifest themselves as tachycardia, hypertension, headache and sweating, and these symptoms account for a substantial number of adverse reactions.

Vasovagal attacks

Vasovagal or syncopal attacks occur very frequently in young subjects. They cause feelings of faintness and, sometimes, loss of consciousness, and they can practically always be diagnosed by the obvious bradycardia.

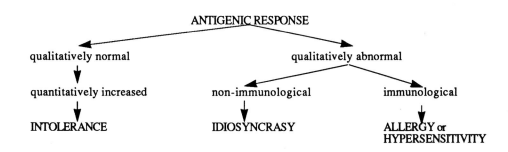

183

Hyperventilation syndrome

Moneret-Vautrin and co-workers (9) have long stressed that the hyperventilation syndrome (or spasmophilia) occurs frequently and that anxiety plays an important part in triggering the crisis. The symptoms are formication (an ant-like, 'crawling' sensation of the skin), malaise and sometimes Trousseau's sign. Milam (10) strongly recommends diazepam sedation to eliminate this as a cause when the differential diagnosis is difficult.

Asthmatic symptoms

These may be caused by the metabisulphite which is added as a preservative to solutions of adrenaline.

Malignant hyperpyrexia

This is very rare, but the amide family of drugs have been incriminated. Some workers (11,12) regard this as justification for the use of procaine in patients at risk from this condition. However, modern opinion favours the use of both ester and amide local anaesthetics (See chapter on Neurological Conditions). The term "allergy" is too often misapplied to the various reactions which may appear when patients have been given local anaesthetics. It should in fact be confined to patients who exhibit specific Ab and/or sensitised lymphocytes.

Allergy to local anaesthetics

The local anaesthetics most commonly used clinically are the amino-amides and amino-esters. There is a third group, with a guanidine-type structure, which has very powerful anaesthetic effects. Tetrodotoxin and saxitonin are examples, but they are not yet on the market. They may be of some importance in the future (7).

Amino-esters

These are derivatives of para-amino-benzoic acid and are characterised by an aromatic lipophilic nucleus, an intermediate ester-linked chain, and a secondary or tertiary amine hydrophilic group. They are hydrolysed in the plasma by pseudocholinesterase. Procaine is a typical example. Ester-based local anaesthetics have long been recognised as a cause of allergies or allergic-type reactions and are best avoided if a suitable amide alternative is available. 2-chloroprocaine in particular has been incriminated.

Methylparahydroxybenzoic acid

The structure of methylparahydroxybenzoic acid or methylparaben is particularly noteworthy. It has an NH_2 radical, like the esters, with which it shares cross-sensitivity. Methylparaben is a preservative with marked bacteriostatic and fungistatic properties and, most important, it is used as a preservative of amide local anaesthetics. Hence, it should always been borne in mind that an allergy presumed to be due to an amide local anaesthetic may in fact be due to this preservative (13). Skin tests for lidocaine and methylparaben must be carried out separately, and a preservative-free solution of lidocaine must of course be used in the lidocaine test. If a patient is known to be allergic to esters, a preservative-free amide local anaesthetic will have to be used (7).

Amino-amides

These consist of an aromatic lipophilic nucleus, an intermediate amide-linked chain and a secondary or tertiary amine hydrophilic group. They are broken down by hepatic enzymes. Lidocaine was the first of this series.

Allergy to amides

This is the subject of debate. Brown (1) described an allergic reaction after the intradermal injection of 0.2ml of 0.5% bupivacaine. There was no local reaction, but the patient felt acutely unwell and developed extensive urticaria. Laboratory tests revealed a minor degree of complement C3 conversion and a marked reduction in complement C4 concentration. The immunoglobulin IgE was not involved in the reaction. Thirty minutes prior to this test, an intradermal injection of 0.2ml of 0.5% prilocaine had been given. This caused a slight skin reaction which faded after 15 minutes. This case seems to be the only one in the literature which is supported by specific immunological investigations.

Fisher (14) reported a case who had previously suffered bronchospasm under lidocaine anaesthesia and who subsequently developed a positive reaction after intradermal injections of very dilute lidocaine and procaine. A similar test for bupivacaine was negative and this drug was used uneventfully.

Intradermal test

The intradermal test is much debated because it is difficult to interpret. Aldrete (15) observed that 40% out of a series of 60 patients with no history of allergy reacted positively to esters, and that this response became negative if an antihistamine was given. However, the response was not modified by antihistamines in patients with a previous history of allergy. The test therefore provides no basis for concluding whether or not a patient is hypersensitive, but merely indicates whether a particular drug can be given. False positive responses might be caused by major histamine release resulting, for example, from needle trauma, tissue distension or additives to the injected drug. The Prausnitz Kustner test is inappropriate (16,17,4,8).

The reliability of the basophil degranulation test is disputed and the conjunctival sensitivity test has already caused one death following the instillation of a drop of local anaesthetic (18).

Allergic or atopic children

Atopy is a familial predisposition in which weak reagins (or Abs) offer little protection.
Atopic conditions include asthma, hay fever and eczema, with pollen, dust, foods or animal hair or fur as the allergens.

There are no formal contraindications to the use of local anaesthetics in atopic, allergic or even frankly asthmatic children. Indeed, these patients may be improved by the reduction in stress which results from freedom from pain. However, for these children and for those who are thought to be allergic to local anaesthetics, certain rules must be followed:

Benzodiazepines should be prescribed as premedication to raise the convulsion threshold (17) and to reduce anxiety which can be a cause of adverse reactions (10).

H1 (e.g. hydroxyzine, diphenhydramine) and H2 (e.g. cimetidine) receptor antagonists may, in association, prevent or reduce the allergic response by occupying peripheral receptor sites. They can be recommended for atopic patients with a history of allergic reaction and for those who are exposed to a second contact with the allergen within a few days of anaesthesia (19).

Intolerance to conventional vasoconstrictors requires that they are withdrawn and replaced, if necessary, by vasopressins such as octapressin (17)(20).

Treatment of allergic reactions

Treatment is essentially supportive. Oxygen and standard resuscitation facilities should be available for the more serious cases. Adrenaline limits the vasoplegic effects of histamine and is the treatment of choice for anaphylactic shock. The effect of diphenhydramine is reduced if the receptor sites are saturated with histamine. Intravenous corticosteroids are often given, but evidence for their beneficial effect is still lacking.

Conclusions

Adverse reactions and allergic mechanisms in response to local anaesthetics are rare, but it is essential that they should not be overlooked when they occur. No case of true hypersensitivity has been described in a child, and before making this diagnosis to explain an acute allergic episode such as Quincke's oedema, generalised urticaria or bronchospasm, it is necessary to exclude other possible causative agents such as antibiotics, acetylsalicylic acid or other anti-inflammatory drugs, and paraben and its derivatives (21).

References

1. Brown DT, Beamish D, Wildsmith JAW (1981) Allergic reactions to an amide local anaesthetic. Br J Anaesth 53:435
2. Giovannitti JA, Bennett CR (1979) Assessment of allergy to local anesthetics. Jada 98:701
3. Aldrete JA, Johnson DA (1970) Evaluation of intracutaneous testing for investigation of allergy to local anesthetic agents. Anesth Analg 49:173
4. Incaudo G, Schatz M, Patterson R, Rosenberg M,

Yamamoto F, Hamburger RN (1978) Administration of local anesthetics to patients with a history of prior adverse reaction.J Allergy Clin Immunol 61:339

5. Foreman JC (1981) The pharmacological control of immediate hypersensitivity. Ann Rev Pharmacol Toxicol 21:63

6. Walton B (1981) Immunological Aspects of Anaesthetic Practice. In "Scientific Foundations of Anaesthesia" 2nd Edition. Heinemann Medical Books Limited

7. Covino BG, Vassallo HG (1976) Local Anesthetics, Mechanisms of Action and Clinical Use. The Scientific Basis of Clinical Anesthesia. Grune & Stratton, Orlando

8. Winnie AP (1984) Plexus Anesthesia Vol 1 p 224. Schultz Copenhagen

9. Moneret-Vautrin DA, Duc M, Sigiel M (1976) Etude de Différents facteurs de risque du déclenchement d'accidents aux anesthésiques et myorelaxants. Ann Anesthésiol Fr 17:165

10. Milam SB, Giovannitti JA, Bright D (1983)Hypersensitivity to amide local anesthetics. Oral Surg 56:593

11. Mather LE, Cousins MJ (1979) Local anesthetics and their current clinical use. Drugs 18:185

12. Ellis FR (1980) Inherited Muscle Disease. Br J Anaesth 52:153

13. Johnson WT (1983) Hypersensitivity to pro-caine, tetracaine, mepivacaine and methylparaben: Report of a case. Jada 106:53

14. Fisher MMcD, Pennington JC (1982) Allergy to local anaesthesia. Br J Anaesth 54:893

15. Aldrete JA, Johnson D (1969) Allergy to local anesthetics. JAMA 207:356

16. Laxenaire MC, Moneret-Vautrin DA, Veryloet D, Alazia M, Francois G (1985) Accidents anaphylactoides graves peranesthésiques. Ann Fr Anesth Réanim 4:30

17. Moneret-Vautrin DA (1985) Les réactions adverses aux anesthésiques locaux. Conceptions actuelles - Stratégies diagnostiques - Aspects préventifs. Allerg et Immunol 17:369

18. Adriani T (1972) Etiology and management of adverse reactions to local anesthetics. Int anesthesiol Clin 10:127

19. Doenicke A, Lorenz W (1982) Histamine release in anaesthesia and surgery. Premedication with H1- and H2- receptor antagonists: indications, benefits and possible problems. Klin Wochenschr 60:1039

20. Aellig WH, O'Neill R, Laurence DR et al. (1970) Cardiac effects of adrenaline and felypressin as vasoconstrictors in local anaesthesia for oral surgery under diazepam sedation. Brit J Anaesth 42:174

21. Schamberg IM (1968) Allergic contact dermatitis to methyl and propyl paraben. Arch Derm 95:626

Coagulopathy

Catherine Esteve

Many authors (1,2,3,4,5,) believe that coagulation disorders rule out completely the use of local and regional anaesthetic techniques. Others (6,7,8,9,) consider that such disorders are only a relative contraindication.

The danger is that blood vessels may be damaged during the performance of the block and that excessive bleeding and haematoma formation may occur. If direct pressure can be applied to the site, the bleeding can be controlled fairly easily, but in the case of deep injections for central blocks, this may not always be feasible. The clinical effect of a haematoma depends on whether the compressed neural tissue is surrounded by bone. For example, compression of the spinal cord may cause paraplegia, and it must be detected and treated without delay - within six hours - if irreversible damage is to be avoided. On the other hand, nerves surrounded by soft tissues are unlikely to be exposed to harmful compression when a haematoma occurs, though the regional technique may well be blamed for the complication.

Epidural haematoma

Epidural haematoma may occur spontaneously in patients who have no coagulation anomalies and who are not receiving anticoagulant treatment (10), but it is well known that such haematomata occur more frequently in the presence of a coagulation disorder (11), even when there has been no precipitating cause, such as a lumbar puncture.

More than one hundred cases of epidural haematoma have been reported in patients who were on anticoagulant therapy, but who had not received a spinal or epidural block (12). It is reasonable to suppose, therefore, that if spinal and epidural blocks were to be performed in these patients, even minor damage to epidural vessels would increase the risk of haematoma.

Subdural haematoma

Subdural haematoma is very rare. Only 20 cases have been reported, and most of these occurred following minor injury or in patients with some coagulation abnormalities (13).

Congenital haemorrhagic disorders

Opinion is that these conditions are absolute contraindications to the use of local and regional techniques (Table 17). However, Hack and colleagues (7) reported 46 patients, between 14 and 50 years of age and suffering from haemophilia A or B, who received spinal or epidural blocks - 35 spinals and 11 con-tinuous epidurals with catheter - for orthopaedic operations on the lower limb. No haematoma occured, but pre-operative evaluation was strict: patients with

Table 17. Coagulation abnormalities

Thromboplastin formation disorders
    a) haemophilia A, B, C.
    b) deficiency in factor X11
    c) Willebrand's disease

Thrombin formation disorders
    deficiencies in factors II, V, V11, X.

Fibrin formation disorders
    a) congenital afibrinogenaemia
    b) dysfibrinogenaemia
    c) factor V111 deficiency

BLOOD PLATELET PATHOLOGY

Thrombocytopaenia due to disorder of medullary production
    a) Fanconi's disease
    b) thrombocytopaenia with absence of
      megakaryocytes
    c) Wiskott-Aldrich syndrome

Thrombocytopathies
    a) Glanzmann's disease
    b) Bernard and Soulier's haemorrhagic
      thrombocyte dystrophy
    c) disorders in the secretory
      function of platelets

factor VIII inhibition were excluded, blood coagulation tests were performed frequently both during and after operation, and factor deficiency was corrected to give a minimal plasma level of 100 %. In view of the risks involved, the use of this technique must be open to question. General anaesthesia gives rise to no particular difficulties in these patients, so it is a safer alternative and it is in any case always required when regional anaesthesia is performed in young children.

Acquired haematological disorders

It is unusual to find children receiving anticoagulant therapy or being treated with long-term acetyl salicylic acid (Aspirin). Nevertheless, these drugs do have clinical relevance and the management of patients receiving them is controversial.

Anticoagulant therapy

The paediatric anaesthetist is rarely confronted with thrombo-embolic disorders, and the question of anticoagulant treatment arises only in special cases, such as an immobilised overweight adolescent or, more commonly, a child with a heart complaint.

De Angelis (16) and Crawford (17) consider that epidural anaesthesia should not be used for patients receiving anticoagulant treatment, but others disagree. Many series have been published in which no complications occurred and the cases reported by van Steenberge and Brichant (18), Odoom and Sih (19) and Rao and El Etr (8) amount in total to over 9.000. However, all these authors took the precaution of excluding patients with congenital and acquired coagulation abnormalities, those with leukaemia and those taking acetyl salicylic acid (Aspirin). They used a midline approach to the epidural space and took great care when introducing the catheter.

The time at which the catheter is withdrawn must be chosen so that anticoagulant activity is minimal: for example, one hour before an injection of heparin is due. The patient should be examined for any abnormal neurological signs at regular intervals and before the administration of top-up doses.

Acetyl salicylic acid therapy

It is well known that some drugs, such as Aspirin, can cause thrombocytopathies. Aspirin brings about a reduction in the second phase of platelet aggregation by inhibiting the release of ADP. Benzon (6) showed that the bleeding time of patients taking Aspirin could be longer than normal, whatever the dose and duration of the treatment. He considered therefore that, when local or regional anaesthesia is planned, the bleeding and clotting times should be measured in all patients taking Aspirin. If a patient with an epidural catheter in place requires anti-pyretic treatment in the post-operative period, it is preferable to use paracetamol rather than Aspirin.

Guidelines for management

A child may require surgery before abnormalities of the coagulation process have made themselves clinically apparent and mild forms of coagulopathy may remain latent. It is advisable to question the parents in detail before deciding on local or regional anaesthesia.

Previously unsuspected disorders may be revealed by pre-operative blood tests which should include activated clotting time, platelet count and prothrombin time. In infants less than 6 months old, coagulation tests may suffice, but if any of these are abnormal, further investigations, including the bleeding time, should be performed.

The possibility of discovering an abnormality leads some anaesthetists, including the author, to perform screening tests on all children for whom regional anaesthesia is planned, but most anaesthetists prefer to reserve these investiga-tions for children in whom there is clinical evidence, or a history, of a coagulation disorder.

Before considering the use of regional anaesthesia in a child whose haemostatic mechanisms are not perfect, the risks must be weighed against the advantages. Only very rarely will the balance be in favour of regional anaesthesia.

Conclusion

An epidural haematoma exerting pressure on the spinal cord causes damage which rapidly becomes irreversible. Although this complication is rare, the possible neurological sequelae, with their medico-legal consequences, mean that any disorder in the haemostatic mechanisms of a child must be carefully investigated. Such disorders are almost always an absolute contra-indication to spinal and epidural anaesthesia. Peripheral regional anaesthetic techniques may be used in such children, but with great caution.

References

1. Gauthier-Lafaye (1985) Précis d'anesthésie loco-régionale. Masson Editeur
2. Lecron L. L'anesthésie péridurale. Encycl Med Chirurgicale Paris. Anesthésie-Réanimation - Fasc 36325 A10
3. Saint-Maurice CI. La rachianesthésie. Encycl Med Chirurgicale Paris. Anesthésie-Réanimation - Fasc 36324 A10
4. Moore Daniel C (1973) Regional Block. Fourth edition. Charles C Thomas Publ,,Springfield
5. Macintosh Sir R (1979) Pratique de la rachianesthésie et de l'anesthésie péridurale. Edition Medsi 4éme edition
6. Benzon H, Brunner E (1984) Bleeding time and nerve blocks after aspirin. Regional anesthesia: Vol 9 n° 2 April-June:86
7. Hack G, Hofmann P, Brackmann HH, Stoeckel H, Pichotka (1980) Erste Erfahrungen mit rücken-marksnahen Regional-anästhesietechniken beim Hämophiliepatienten: Anästh Intensivther Notfallimed 15:45
8. Rao TLK, El Etr AA (1981) Anticoagulation following placement of epidural and subarachnoid catheters. An evaluation of neurologic sequelae. Anesthesiology 55:618
9. Van Steenberge A (1969) L'anesthésie péridurale. Masson Editeur
10. Markham JW, Lynge HN (1967) The syndrome of spontaneous spinal epidural hematoma. J of Neurosurg 26:334
11. Sreerama VI, Dennery JM (1973) Neurosurgical complications of anticoagulant therapy. Canad Med Assoc J 108:305
12. Cousins MJ (1972) Hematoma following epidural block. Anesthesiology 37:263
13. Greensite FS, Katz J (1980) Spinal subdural hematoma associated with attempted epidural anesthesia and subsequent continuous spinal anesthesia: Anesthesia and Analgesia 59, 1
14. Aitkenhead AR, Grant IS (1983) Interactions with concurrent disease medication, in Practical Regional Anesthesia. Edited by JJ Henderson and WS Nimmo. Chapt 7:143
15. Mattei, Orsini A (1982) Hématologie pédiatrique. Flammarion Médecine-Sciences. Chapt. 22:320
16. De Angelis J (1976) Hazards of subdural and epidural anesthesia during anticoagulant therapy: a case report and review. Anesth Analg 5:293
17. Crawford JS(1975) Pathology in extradural space. BJA 47:412
18. Van Steenberge A, Brichant JF (1985) Anesthesie loco-règionale et traitemzent anticoagulant: Choisir le risque. IVème Journèes de Mise au Point en Anesthèsie Rèanimation MAPAR Editions 445
19. Odoom JA, Sih LI (1983) Epidural analgesia and anticoagulant therapy. Experience with one thousand cases of continuous epidurals. Anaesthesia 38:254

Myopathy

Jean-Luc Hody, Catherine Estève

The term myopathy covers a wide range of diseases of striated muscle, characterised by progressive muscle fibre degeneration. Progressive myopathies share in common the fact that at the outset the disorder is confined to certain muscles, but is subsequently found throughout the entire muscular system.

In general, myopathies can be classified as primary or secondary. The former group includes muscular dystrophies, congenital myopathies and metabolic myopathies. The latter covers conditions arising from spinal cord disease, peripheral nervous disorders and disorders of the neuromuscular junction (myasthenia).

This chapter will be mainly concerned with the muscular dystrophies, which can be divided into four groups. A brief description of Groups II, III and IV will be given first, followed by a more detailed description of Duchenne's disease which is the most dramatic form of muscular dystrophy and accounts for 80% of all hereditary muscular diseases.

Fig. 122.

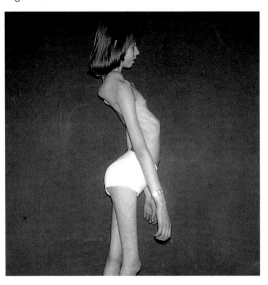

Muscular dystrophies

Dystrophies with recessive autosomal transmission (Gr. II)
Of the girdle types of muscular dystrophy, the pelvifemoral (Leyden Moebius) occurs more frequently than the scapulohumeral (Erb). The disease progresses slowly and is variable in its stages of development. It may begin between the first and third decades of life.

Dystrophies with dominant autosomal transmission (Gr. III)
This group includes facioscapulohumeral dystrophy (Landouzy Dejerine disease). It progresses very slowly and is essentially asymmetrical.

Myotonic dystrophies with dominant autosomal transmission (Gr. IV)
The most prevalent form is Steinert's disease in which the child usually shows severe symptoms of hypotonia and respiratory distress at birth.

Progressive muscular dystrophy or Duchenne muscular dystrophy (D.M.D)
This condition, also known as Duchenne de Boulogne's disease or DDB 1, is the most common form of myopathy and the best known. There has been little to add to Duchenne's clinical description since his original publication in 1868 (1).

Clinical appearance diagnosis and prognosis

This recessive, sex-linked disease, which only affects boys, has an incidence of 0.14 per 1000 children. It usually commences at about 18 months with an excessive tendency to fatigue, first in walking and then in climbing stairs. Hypertrophy of the calves becomes apparent. This is a pseudohypertrophy and the increase in muscle mass soon gives way to fatty infiltration.

Obesity is common, and the condition gets

progressively worse. 75% of patients die before the age of 20 years, death being due to chronic respiratory insufficiency in 50% of cases, acute cardio-respiratory insufficiency (30%), cardiac insufficiency (10%) or heart rate disorders (10%) (Fig. 123) (2).

Major functional disorders

These are always the direct or indirect result of the muscular atrophy which the disease causes. Lingual hypertrophy and the respiratory and cardiac pathology make these cases a challenge to the anaesthetist.

Surgical aspects

Apart from emergency operations for acute abdominal pain and tracheostomies for assisted ventilation, surgery is most commonly performed on the lower limbs and spinal column. Current opinion favours surgical intervention

Fig. 123. Muscular degeneration (Courtery of Dr Ph Soudon).

earlier and earlier in the course of the disease so that the patient's ability to stand and walk can be extended (3,4). Anaesthesia for these procedures should be as light as possible (5,6,7).

Anaesthetic aspects

In the pre-operative examination, the anaesthetist must take into account the respiratory muscle weakness which results in alveolar hypo-ventilation, microatelectasis, reduced coughing power and the restrictive syndrome, giving a dramatically low vital capacity. Scoliosis may contribute to ventilation- perfusion problems, and regurgitation and pulmonary aspiration may occur. In addition, cardiomyopathy and heart rate disorders may be present and there is also a risk of malignant hyperpyrexia (8,9,10), hyper-kalaemia and rhabdomyolysis (11, 12).

The surgeon, guided by his desire to improve the quality of life for these children, often wishes to carry out a wide range of operations with the result that the anaesthetist is asked to accept

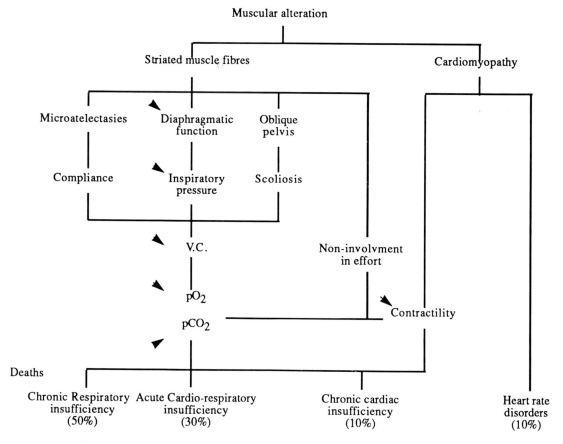

patients who are very bad anaesthetic risks.

Premedication should be avoided where possible, but if it is essential, the rectal or oral route is preferred. Diazepam by mouth, or trimeprazine tartrate ($2mg.kg^{-1}$), may be suitable. The preoperative visit is obviously important since it may be just as effective as premedication and may eliminate the need for pre-operative drugs. Anticholinergics are not usually necessary, but should the need arise, hyoscine is preferred to atropine because it causes less tachycardia (5, 13).

Regional anaesthesia

General anaesthesia for cases of muscular dystrophy poses many problems of which the pulmonary handicap is the most important. Regional anaesthesia is therefore the preferred technique (5,6,14,15,16,17) because it does not cause central respiratory depression, and it provides protection against the stress response, supplies postoperative analgesia and permits early passive physiotherapy. With the exception of spinal procedures, which call for general anaesthesia, most operations are on the lower limbs to prolong walking, to facilitate nursing, to prevent bed-sores, postural defects or pelvic obliquity, and for this type of surgery, regional anaesthesia is very suitable.

Special considerations

Obesity
This is particularly common in DMD patients and may make landmarks difficult to feel. The bilateral adipose swellings overlying the paravertebral muscles result in a midline channel being formed between the swellings. When the child is in the lateral decubitus position, this channel tends to slip downwards and may no longer occupy the midline. This can be misleading for identification of the vertebral spines and deep palpation may be required to locate them. Fat may make insertion of intravenous catheters difficult, and limitation of movement of the neck, shoulder and arm, due to muscle contractures and fat, may complicate brachial plexus blocks.

The patient must be handled and placed on the operating table with great care, and pressure points must be protected so that bed-sores are not allowed to develop due to faulty positioning.

Deformities of the spinal column
At the cervical and lumbar level, these may give rise to difficulties with regional anaesthesia. The deformities most frequently encountered are scoliosis with a single curve and dorsolumbar kyphosis. Double curves, lumbar kyphoses with the back flat and even unfixed hyperlordoses also occur. In the post-pubertal myopathic patient with severe contractures, these large hyperlordoses are fixed and access between the vertebral spines becomes very difficult. Vertebral rotation is apparent from the onset of the condition and increases with it. It is usually most marked at the L1 - 2 level where it may reach nearly 50° It is sometimes necessary for the anaesthetist to resort to the paramedian route for epidural or spinal anaesthesia when he is confronted by these deformities.

Per-operative management
Cardiac and respiratory rate, arterial pressure, oxygen saturation and % CO_2 are monitored by non-invasive methods. Insertion of a thermometer is recommended for regular temperature monitoring. For longer operations, a urinary catheter is passed. A nasogastric tube serves no purpose because the swallowing reflexes and intestinal motility are retained and oral feeding is quickly resumed. Intravenous fluids should be administered with great care in case the right side of the heart is overloaded.

Fig. 124. Obesity in DMD

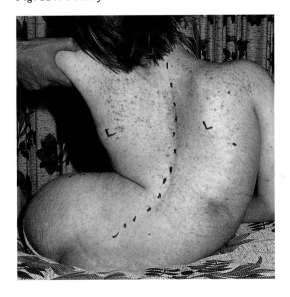

Sedation

Unsupplemented regional anaesthesia is not always possible because the myopathic patient has his own particular mental attitude. He is overprotected, and is often emotional and anxious. Although there are young children whose confidence can be gained in a few hours and with whom it is possible to have an animated conversation, not all children have the same level of self-control. Light sedation will then be required.

The benzodiazepines seem to be a good choice. Flunitrazepam or midazolam may be given as an adjunct to a ketamine infusion when they reduce the cardiostimulating effect of the ketamine (18). Flunitrazepam may also be combined with thalamonal (a mixture of fentanyl and droperidol). These adjuvants give a measure of disassociation and they provide analgesia for all areas not included in the regional block. Patients tend to become restless because they find the operating table uncomfortable. This combination of disassociation and analgesia amounts to a state of hypnoanalgesia (19), which may be defined as a mixture of analgesia and sedation resembling normal sleep or hypnosis, as compared with narcoanalgesia, which is a combination of analgesia and very light, supplemental general anaesthesia or narcosis.

Fig. 125. Deformities in a spinal column.

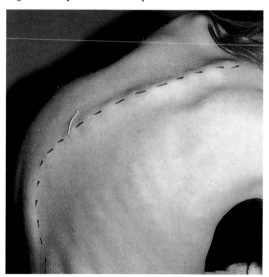

Types of regional anaesthesia

Brachial plexus block
Various forms of brachial plexus block may be performed for upper limb surgery, the axillary route being the most frequently used. It should be borne in mind, as mentioned above, that tendon contractures and obesity may make the techniques difficult, and a nerve stimulator is therefore recommended.

Intravenous regional anaesthesia
In Miller's opinion (13), this should be the ideal technique for the myotonic patient undergoing limb surgery when relaxation is required. However, there are no reports on this subject.

Femoral nerve block
Berkowitz and Rosenberg (20) reported a series of 103 femoral nerve blocks with mepivacaine for muscle biopsy in patients from 4 to 20 years of age likely to develop malignant hyperthermia, and this is certainly a valuable approach.

Spinal anaesthesia
There are no reports in the literature of the use of spinal anaesthesia in myopathic children. A major disadvantage is the short duration of action and the inability to prolong analgesia into the postoperative period without inserting a catheter - a procedure which is still the subject of debate in elderly healthy adults and which is not generally accepted.

Epidural anaesthesia
The practicality of this technique may be limited by obesity of the myopathic patient and by his spinal deformities and rotations.

Caudal anaesthesia
This is the preferred technique for surgery of the lower limb because, at the time when such surgery is being considered, the anatomy is relatively normal and the children have not at that stage developed major sacral canal deformities. For this reason, it is permissible to insert a catheter high up the epidural space as far as it will run, to the lumbar or lower thoracic region for abdominal surgery.

Hody and co-workers (17) have reported on a series of 51 DMD patients who received 65 anaesthetics involving the lower limb. 15 were for changes of plaster or dressings, but the remainder were for surgical procedures involving, in all, 406 different operative sites. Caudal anaesthesia was given in 64,5 %, epidural blocks in 17% and caudal anaesthesia with a very light supplementary general anaesthetic in 11% of these cases.

Choice of local anaesthetic and additives

Lidocaine
In Miller's view (13), this is a good choice for intravenous regional anaesthesia in neuromuscular dystrophies, but Ellis (21) advises against it because of its stimulant effect on muscle.

Prilocaine
This and other ester-linked local anaesthetics have been recommended for patients susceptible to malignant hyperthermia. However, the Professional Advisory Council of the Malignant Hyperthermia Association has recently made a formal statement: "Based on limited clinical and laboratory evidence all local anaesthetic drugs appear to be safe for MH-susceptible individuals".

Bupivacaine
Bupivacaine is still the most commonly used local anaesthetic. The pharmacokinetics of bupivacaine injected by the lumbar epidural route are identical to those reported in normal healthy children of similar age (22).

Fentanyl
Fentanyl may be added to the local anaesthetic and given in a dose of 1 microgram per kg body weight.

Conclusion
By virtue of the advantages which it offers (23), regional anaesthesia is becoming the preferred type of anaesthesia for the myopathic child. It ensures a remarkably high degree of postoperative comfort and allows early physiotherapy for these patients.

References
1. Duchenne de Boulogne (1868) Recherches sur la paralysie musculaire pseudohypertrophique ou paralysie myosclérosique. Archives Gen de Méd (6 sér) 11
2. Soudon Ph, Wouters A, Kulakowski S (1984) PO_2-PCO_2 transcutaneous monitoring during sleep and ventilatory function. Cardiomyology Vol IIi 4:32
3. Dubousset J, Queneau P (1983) Place et indication de la chirurgie dans la dystrophie musculaire de DDB: à évolution rapide. Revue de Chirurgie Orthopédique 69:207
4. Bellen P (1982) Le traitement chirurgical des séquelles de la myopathie. Acta Orthop Belg 48:291
5. Yamashita M, Matsuki A, Oyama T (1976) General anesthesia for a patient with progressive muscular dystrophy. Anaesthesist 25:76
6. Cobham IG, Hamilton SD (1964) Anaesthesia for muscle dystrophy patients. Anesth & Analg 43:22
7. Katz J, Kadis LB (1973) Anesthesia and uncommon disease: pathophysiologic and clinical correlations. 425. Saunders, Philadelphia
8. Brownell AKW, Paasuke RT, Elash A, Fowlow SB, Seagram CGF, Diewold RJ, Friesen C (1983) Malignant hyperthermia in Duchenne muscular dystrophy Anesthesiology 58:150
9. Rosenberg H, Heiman-Patterson T (1983) Duchennés muscular dystrophy and malignant hyperthermia: another warning. Anesthesiology 59:362
10. Kelfer HM, Singler WD, Reynolds RN (1983) Malignant hyperthermia in a child with Duchenne muscular dystrophy. Pediatrics 71:118
11. Miller ED, Sanders DB, Rowlingson JC, Berry FA, Sussman MD, Epstein RM (1978) Anesthesia-induced rhabdomyolysis in a patient with Duchenne's muscular dystrophy. Anesthesiology 48:146
12. Lewandoski K (1981) Rhabdomyolysis, myoglobinuria and hyperpyrexia caused by suxamethonium in a child with increased serum kinase concentration. Br J Anaesth 53:981
13. Miller J, Lee C (1981) Muscle Disease: Anaesthesia and uncommon diseases. Edited by Katz & Benumof. Saunders Co. Philadelphia
14. Kaufman L (1960) Anaesthesia in dystrophia myotonica. Proc Roy Soc Med 53:183
15. Kepes E, Martinez L, Andrew SC (1972) Anesthetic problems in hereditary muscular abnormalities. N.Y. State J Med 1:1051
16. Hody JL (1982) Les problèmes posés par

l'anesthésie du myopathe. Acta Orth Belg 48:302

17. Hody JL (1988) Regional anesthesia in myopathic children. Acta Anaesth Belg 39, 3 suppl 2:209

18. White P (1982) Ketamine: its pharmacology and therapeutic uses. Anesthesiology 56:119

19. Hody JL (1981) Epidural anesthesia for orthopedic surgery. Survey of 730 cases. Sedation and supplementation. Acta Anaesth Belg 32:213

20. Berkowitz A, Rosenberg H (1985) Femoral block with mepivacaine for muscle biopsy in malignant hyperthermia patients. Anesthesiology 62:651

21. Ellis FR (1980) Inherited muscle disease. Br J Anaesth 52:153

22. Murat I, Estéve C, Montay G, Delleur MM, Gaudiche O, Saint-Maurice C (1987) Pharmacokinetics and cardiovascular effects of bupivacaine during epidural anesthesia in children with Duchenne Muscular Dystrophy. Anesthesiology 67:249

23. Spear RM, Deshpande JK, Maxwell LG (1988) Caudal anesthesia in the awake, high-risk infant. Regional Anesthesia 13, 2:24

Index

A

Absorption 9, 46,55, 57, 80, 151
Acidosis 53-54
Action potential 26, 42
    mechanism of 42
Adrenaline 9, 10, 28, 34, 44, 45, 55, 57, 68, 69,
    78, 84, 91, 94-96, 100, 104, 108, 109, 116,
    117, 122, 124, 129, 151, 153, 157, 160,
    170, 173, 182, 183, 185
Airway management 178
Albumin 52, 56
Allergy 50, 63, 183
Alpha 1-acid glycoprotein 52
amethocaine 122
Amide 40, 50, 184
Anatomical difference 9, 16
Anatomy,
    dorsal nerve of the penis 157
    femoral nerve 140
    ilio-hypogastric nerve 155
    ilioinguinal nerve 155
    lateral cutaneous nerve 141
    obturator nerve 142
    perineal nerve 157
    posterior cutaneous nerve of the thigh 141
    sacral hiatus 83
    sciatic nerve 143, 146
    spine 17
    sural nerve 147
    tibial nerve 145-147
Ankle block 146
Apnoea 11, 34, 179
Arnold Chiari syndrome 18
Aspiration test 84, 94, 104, 108, 116
Aspirin 188
Autonomic reflex 11
Axillary catheter 175
    approach 133

B

Baroreflex 33
Benefits 11, 34
Beta-endorphine 31
Biliary surgery 114
Bioavailability 46
Bleeding 11, 187, 188
Block failure 66
    frequency dependent 43

Blood flow, regional 34
    patch 104
    vessels puncture 70, 86, 105
Body temperature 52
Brachial plexus block 14
    axillary 64, 133, 169, 175
    continous 175
    interscalene 130
    perivascular subclavian 132
    supraclavicular 128, 130
Bronchoscopy 161
Buck´s fascia 158
Bupivacaine 9, 11, 28, 29, 41, 43-49, 50-53, 55,
    78-81, 83, 95, 100, 108, 109, 114, 117, 121,
    122, 125, 128, 139, 141, 142, 145-147, 151,
    153, 154, 156, 158, 159, 169-171, 174, 176,
    185, 194

C

Calcium channel blockers 56
Carbonated local anaesthetics 43
Cardiac arrest 44
    depression 44
    output 52
Cardio toxicity 43
Catheter technique 69-71, 88
Caudal block 14, 34, 55, 69, 81, 88, 166, 174,
    179
Central nervous system 17
Cerebral palsy 180
Cerebro spinal fluid 21, 119
    spinal volume 21
Cervical rib 19
Chemical neurolysis 173, 175
Children information 60, 61
Chloroprocaine 50, 126, 128, 182, 184
Choroid plexus 21
Chronic pain 173-177
Cimetidine 56, 185
Cinchocaine 122
Circumcision 83, 168, 179
Clearance 46, 49, 51, 151
CNS toxicity 43, 53
CO_2 response 118, 170
Coagulation abnormalities 10, 64, 78, 187
Coarctation of aorta 114
Coelio-splanchnic block 175
Column development 18
Compliance 29
Complication of RA 11, 33, 63, 67, 85, 96,
    103, 105, 108, 111, 118, 124, 129, 152,
    156, 157, 160, 162, 164, 167, 179

G

General anaesthesia 8, 10, 11, 13, 14, 32-34, 36, 37, 56, 61, 63-68, 78, 83, 91, 95, 101, 107, 108, 110, 112-115, 117, 119, 124-127, 146, 156-158,160-161, 166, 178-80, 188, 192-193

H

Haemodynamic effect 32, 34
    lumbar blocks 32, 168
    spinal block 32
    thoracic block 32, 117
Halothane 11, 13, 33, 34, 36, 45, 62, 66, 119, 158
Headache 67, 104, 124
Hepatectomy 114
Hepatic clearance 51
    bloodflow 56
Hernia incarcerated 11, 81
    repair 81, 124, 156, 168, 179
Hyperbaric solution 121, 122
Hypospadias 81
Hypotension 11, 13, 33, 34, 36, 45, 62, 66, 119, 158, 175
Hypovolaemia 78

I

Ilio-hypogastric nerve 155
    block 155
Ilioinguinal nerve 155
    block 155, 168
Implantable reservoir 174
Infusion pump 174
Inguinal hernia (incarcerated) 81
Interaction of local anaesthetics
    with premedication 56
    with general anaesthesia 56
    with other medications 56
Intercostal
    block 55, 149, 169, 175
    catheter 175
    muscle 149
    nerve 149
Intrapleural
    catheter 153, 169
    regional anaesthesia 153
Intravenous regional anaesthesia 159, 176
Intraventricular catheter 174
Intussusception 99
Ionisation 41

K

Ketamine 66, 67, 78, 83, 121, 124, 158, 193
Klippel-Feil syndrome 19

L

Lateral cutaneous nerve block 141
Level of blockade (test) 62, 65, 66, 91
Lidocaine 42-44, 50-55, 57, 78, 79, 83, 89, 91, 100, 110, 121, 122, 126, 128, 143, 145-147, 151, 159, 161, 163, 164, 175, 182-184
Ligamentum flavum 22, 102-104, 111, 112, 115
Liposolubility 40-42
Local anaesthetic, see drug
Loss of resistance 103, 115
Lumbar epidural block 98
Lung uptake 49

M

Magendi foramen 21
Malignant hyperthermia 11, 64, 182, 184
Management 63
Mechanism of action 26, 42
Median nerve block 135
Medicolegal aspect 61, 180
Mepivacaine 41, 50-52, 54, 78, 82, 83, 89, 91, 95, 100, 110, 126, 128, 143, 145-147, 193
Metabolism 44-50
Methaemoglobinaemia 44, 164
Mixture of LA 56
Modulated receptor hypothesis 43
Monitoring 10, 65
Morphine 57, 151, 167, 169-171, 174
Multiple sclerosis 181
Muscle relaxation 11
Myasthenia gravis 182
Myelinisation 28, 42
Myopathy 190

N

Naloxone 57, 170
Narcotics 57, 174
Nausea 57, 170
Neck 18
Needle see equipment
Nephrectomy 114
Nerve (see also anatomy)
    conduction 28
    damage 180